Peplau's Model
in Action

The Roper–Logan–Tierney Model in Action
C. NEWTON

Peplau's Model in Action
H. SIMPSON

Orem's Model in Action
S. CAVANAGH

Further Models in preparation

Riehl's Model in Action
Neumann's Model in Action

Peplau's Model in Action

HOWARD SIMPSON

BA, M.Ed., Dip. Ed., SRN, RMN, RNT
District Psychiatric Education Centre,
Mapperley Hospital,
Nottingham

Series Editor
BOB PRICE

BA, M.Sc., SRN, Cert. Ed. (Education)
Army Medical Services School of Nursing,
Woolwich

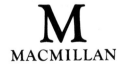

MACMILLAN

First published 1991 by
THE MACMILLAN PRESS LTD
Houndmills, Basingstoke, Hampshire RG21 2XS
and London
Companies and representatives
throughout the world

Designed by Claire Brodmann

ISBN 0–333–52323–7

A catalogue record for this book is available
from the British Library

Printed in Great Britain by
Billing and Sons Ltd
Worcester

Reprinted 1992

CONTENTS

Certain conventions have been observed in the writing of this book. First, a person receiving nursing care is usually referred to as a 'patient', but in some contexts as a 'client'; the terms are often interchangeable and their use tends to be dictated by local practice. Secondly, although people in the book are introduced with their full names and titles they are usually referred to thereafter by their first name only – this reflects the trust established in effective nurse–patient relationships; each patient is understood to have consented to this use of his or her name. Thirdly, unless the context requires otherwise the nurse is referred to as 'she' and the patient as 'he'. These conventions are solely for reasons of simplicity, clarity and style.

A major move in the last few years has been from a medical model of care to a nursing model. As one of the *Nursing Models in Action* series, Peplau's developmental nursing model uses as its main theme the skill of interaction. Experienced nurses all say that caring for someone involves both doing things for him and being able to relate to the person. In writing this book Howard Simpson has identified aspects of Peplau's model that are important concepts to understand and use in practice.

Part I of the book looks at the model as it can be used today. This part of the book is designed for nurses in a basic educational programme, for those learning about different models, for nurses who wish to return to practice, and for readers who wish to look at the Peplau model in greater depth.

Part II of the book considers the application of Peplau's model in practice and draws on five patient dependency studies both within and outside hospital. This section encourages the reader to see the potential use of Peplau in a variety of nursing situations and is designed to help stimulate discussion through the questions and exercises provided.

Part III of the book provides a critique of the Peplau model, aimed at helping the reader to see where the potential and the weaknesses of such a model lie. Readers are encouraged to look at this model in an informed way; it is hoped that they will come to their own decision about its use in today's nursing world.

Throughout the book, particularly in the final part, the author has put his own interpretation on some aspects of Peplau's model. This has been done to help the reader assess the applicability of the original concepts, ideas and values put forward by Peplau to an actual nursing system. In the case of this author the system is the

British nursing system, but the book will be relevant to many other parts of the world, and the reader may find principles of application that will help in adapting Peplau's model to other nursing systems.

The sections on 'The use of counselling skills' and 'Providing a network of support for staff' in Chapter 9 are included by the author to help the reader to think about the implementation of Peplau's model in different care settings; they are therefore adjuncts to the discussion about the use of the model in hospital and community settings, and to the original thoughts of Peplau, recorded in her book, *Interpersonal Relations in Nursing*.

Bob Price

ACKNOWLEDGEMENTS

I would particularly like to thank Hildegard Peplau for her help and support in the writing of this book.

I would also like to thank my family and the many colleagues and friends who have given me constructive advice. Special thanks go to Bob Price for his help; and to Pat Bateman, who typed the manuscript.

Howard Simpson

The author and publishers have made every effort to trace copyright holders, but if any have been overlooked the publishers will be pleased to make the necessary arrangements at the first opportunity.

PART I

Peplau's model today

CHAPTER ONE

The nature of Peplau's developmental model

Those concerned with caring for people who are ill are frequently confronted with the problem of how to provide the highest quality of care in the most proficient and cost-effective way. As part of this health care, nurses today are looking at suitable frameworks in which to practise, and thereby be able to assist the patient or client to full recovery, or to an assisted independence, or to a peaceful death.

This book is about one such framework, Peplau's developmental model of nursing care, and its potential application in a variety of health-care settings. In principle, a model can be useful only if it can be put into practice sensibly and dynamically, preferably with a minimum of jargon. It has to be seen as a useful device or tool which nurses can value and identify with, and which therefore provides them with a knowledge structure to enable care to be organised in a realistic and systematic way. In short, nurses should be able to use a model that supports their practice and in doing so helps direct their thinking, feeling and doing. Peplau's model is designed to assist nurses to understand aspects of the nurse–patient relationship; it also suggests guides for action.

In writing about the model, Peplau saw the cornerstone of success as the establishment and nurturing of the nurse–patient relationship. Without this, the nurse could not really be helpful and therapeutic, and the process of care would therefore be ineffective. The dynamics of the interaction between nurse and patient in exploring and understanding the patient's needs, feelings, attitudes and beliefs, as well as those of the nurse, were seen as vital in providing a partnership in caring with the patient.

Peplau saw the nurse–patient relationship as developing through interlocking or overlapping phases of interaction. These phases occur, whether or not they are recognised; the question is whether

1

the nurse is aware of the particular phase of the nurse–patient relationship operative at a given time, of the particular requirements, and of the readiness of the patient to move towards the next phase. For this awareness to be achieved the nurse needs to have a clear understanding of how and what she communicates with the patient. In addition she needs to think carefully about her nursing knowledge, her own beliefs about caring, and her attitude towards care.

THE ORIGIN OF PEPLAU'S MODEL

The publication in 1952 of Hildegard Peplau's book on *Interpersonal Relations in Nursing* brought into being a theoretical framework in which nurses could look systematically at the care they gave, particularly in the field of mental health nursing. In particular, her theory looked at the importance of the nurse–patient relationship, and her ideas about nursing were drawn from the concepts of personal, developmental and interpersonal skills and learning theory. In her original work, Peplau described her model as a 'partial theory for the practice of nursing': in this sense, she saw the care given to patients as a developing type of care in which trusting relationships formed the basis of successful outcomes.

Peplau saw illness as a potential learning experience. Through the development of a meaningful nurse–patient relationship both the patient and nurse would learn, grow and develop themselves further as persons. Peplau asserted that for nurses to achieve effective care they would need to develop and mature as individuals in their own right; as a result the patient would have a greater opportunity to learn from the nurse about his illness, so gaining a greater insight into himself and his present condition. Once this situation had been recognised and achieved, the patient could begin to manage his feelings and actions in relation to his health problems. These considerations in turn affect her skill in applying her knowledge of nursing to particular patients. In the introduction to her original book (Peplau 1952, p. xii), Peplau talks about her first guiding assumption: that the patient is better cared for if the nurse is more aware of herself. She states: 'the kind of person each nurse becomes makes a substantial difference in what the patient will learn as he is nursed throughout his experience with others'. This statement enables us to consider Peplau's framework for nursing:

2

fostering personality development in the direction of maturity is a function of nursing and nursing education; it requires the use of principles and methods that permit and guide the process of grappling with everyday interpersonal problems or difficulties.

HEALTH AND ILL HEALTH

Peplau considered that health is 'a symbol that implies a forward movement of personality and other on-going human processes in a direction of creative, constructive, productive personal and community living' (Peplau 1988, p. 12). For Peplau health is a concept, a quality which is dynamic, allowing a person the potential experience of physical and social well-being, and giving that person an opportunity to live well and in harmony with others.

Peplau also sees the process of nursing as goal-directed: it requires a series of actions to help the patient move towards achieving health. The nurse–patient relationship is essentially the setting in which the beliefs, values, attitudes and knowledge of the patient and nurse can be used to explore and understand the dynamics of healthy living.

The question to be asked at this juncture is this: 'Is the promotion of health a realistic or true goal of nursing?' In some ways, this is a hard question to answer, because nurses tend to work in environments that are essentially illness-orientated, and as a result their thought processes as professionals are often geared towards this line of thinking. How soon do nurses introduce concepts of health to patients? Is it functionally possible always to promote health with all people?

Not all patients are able to be educated towards health because of the limited contact time that nurses have – for example in an accident department, or because the patient is not amenable to the promotion of health, as would be the case with a young child or a confused elderly person. Having said this, though, it is right to assume that nursing practice (as well as medical practice) is aimed at helping the patient in the direction of health.

It is important to see that the processes involved in health, as outlined by Peplau, are processes that nurses can understand and work with in various health-care settings. Nurses therefore need to think of health as a dynamic force, something that is always changing. It influences the decisions they make when organising the overall plan of care. The nurse has to think about how the patient can best put health into practice, to consider what each patient needs in the way of teaching, and to question how prepared she herself is to promote changes in people so that health can be achieved. Peplau suggests that patients can be helped to look at new coping strategies to promote health if the nurse is able to interact effectively and has good knowledge of health issues. The important point is for the nurse to work *with* as well as *for* the patient in order to achieve changes.

Peplau saw that health can fail for a number of reasons:

1 because of a lack of knowledge within the patient, the professionals, and the society in which the patient lives;
2 because a patient has been ill for so long that he or she is incapable of thinking healthily any more without extensive, long-term professional help;
3 because the provision for health is restricted by limited resources – the patient's limited resources, the nurse's limited knowledge, the society's limited financial resources;
4 because of the inability of the health professionals to organise themselves properly, and hence their inability to effectively evoke or create changes in people;
5 because of a poor working relationship between the nurse and the patient.

By addressing these issues, Peplau felt, health could be achieved. Specifically, however, she believed that if a person's illness was well understood by a nurse, and if the nurse had the necessary interpersonal skills to help the person communicate his feelings and thoughts so as to identify gaps in his information and abilities, then there would be a greater chance of promoting health and the general feeling of well-being.

THE NATURE OF MAN

Peplau says of man that he is 'an organism that lives in an unstable equilibrium and life is the process of striving in the direction of stable equilibrium, i.e. a fixed pattern that is never reached except in death'. She saw the function of a person's personality as being to develop and grow, and that of nursing as being a nurturing process that seeks to provide support for this growth and development. The needs of man require nurses to support him in retaining or achieving

4

maximum potential to function independently within a society which influences his growth and maturation as a human being.

Peplau sees this as a primary duty of any nurse. The capacity of a person to develop demands that social processes be considered – education, religion, family, community, friends, social institutions and agencies. Nursing someone involves looking at care in the context of man's needs; nursing is not culture-free. Each person must be seen in the context of his culture and beliefs, for man has not only physical needs, but psychological and social needs as well.

The needs of man are seen as acquired by being born and by living. Peplau raises several points for our consideration of human needs: how are needs expressed? What happens when needs are not met? How do patients demonstrate to nurses that their needs have been met? Do nurses need to take serious notice of all a patient's needs?

Needs are expressed by people when they seek some end result for themselves. When people have their needs satisfied, they grow and develop as human beings, enabling them to seek in a more mature way for further needs to be met. Peplau recognises that needs create tension in someone, and that the behaviour shown by that person is designed to demonstrate and help reduce the tension. Behaviour therefore is seen as an outward expression of the person's needs. When someone is expressing one particular need, the behaviour is simply focused in an attempt to meet that need, to the partial or total exclusion of other needs.

Success in coping with ill health is dependent upon how well a person integrates with the society he comes from; the person has a tendency to withdraw from society when ill in order to help his recovery process. Once well again he rejoins society with all that is demanded of him. Peplau looks at man and how he learns from previous experiences, which in turn influences his perception about being ill and his ability to adapt to being ill. She also sees the need for nurses to observe the nature of the different demands of the patient, especially his dependency on the nurse and how he can learn how to cope with his reactions to illness. It is in the nature of man to behave differently when ill as opposed to being well; it follows that a patient's thinking and feeling about being ill will influence his own behaviour, as will the response of others in his environment. It is often the nurse who is the professional who observes this behaviour and who can use it, to help the patient come to terms with what is happening in his life.

Definition of nursing

In her original work, Peplau summarises the concept of nursing as follows:

> Nursing is a significant, therapeutic, interpersonal process. It functions co-operatively with other human processes that make health possible for individuals in communities. In specific situations in which a professional health team offers health services, nurses participate in the organisation of conditions that facilitate natural on-going tendencies in human organisations. Nursing is an educative instrument, a maturing force, that aims to promote forward movement of personality in the direction of creative, constructive, productive personal and community living.　　　　　　　(Peplau 1988, p. 16)

This summary says a great deal about the potential complexity of nursing and what is required of nurses to ensure that the concept can actually become real in practice. In order to explore the definition of nursing put forward by Peplau, it is helpful to look at the role of a nurse.

Roles of the nurse

Peplau considers carefully the role of the nurse and how this helps the patient to cope with illness and to get better.

A prerequisite to successfully caring for a patient is for the nurse to be a warm person who is skilled in what she does. This is very important, as the nurse–patient relationship is one in which each grows with the other. In this sense Peplau sees nursing as being both 'educative' and 'therapeutic'. Nurses need to be aware of the roles they are taking, or the roles thrust onto them by the patients they nurse. Equally important is being aware of the short- and long-term consequences of these roles for the patients, and of the transition from one role to another, with nurses choosing which role is appropriate at any given time.

In the early stages of a relationship, the nurse needs to ensure that she grasps the present state of understanding that the patient has about his condition, and whether and in what ways she needs to be a knowledgable practitioner for him. Society expects nurses to be authoritative regarding nursing knowledge and practice, so it is important for nurses to decide what roles in nursing actually mean to them, especially as the nurse–patient relationship is so dynamic and experimental. For example, as the relationship with a patient deepens, a nurse can recognise the surrogate roles she may have to

6

Figure 1.1 The development of the nurse–patient relationship (Adapted from Figure 2, 'A continuum showing changing aspects of nurse–patient relations', in Peplau 1988, p. 10)

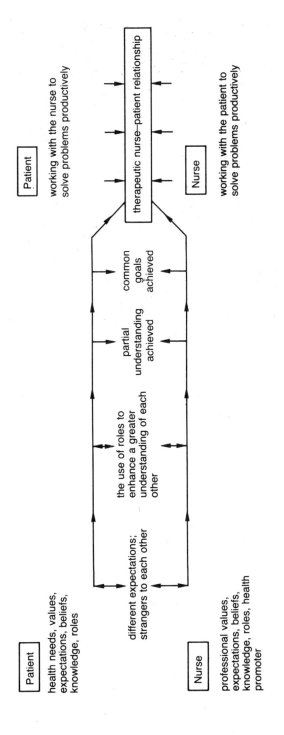

Patient

health needs, values, expectations, beliefs, knowledge, roles

Nurse

professional values, expectations, beliefs, knowledge, roles, health promoter

different expectations; strangers to each other

the use of roles to enhance a greater understanding of each other

partial understanding achieved

common goals achieved

therapeutic nurse–patient relationship

Patient

working with the nurse to solve problems productively

Nurse

working with the patient to solve problems productively

perform – for example as a mother, a sister, a child, an adult – and consider whether or not taking on such roles would be beneficial for the patient in the short and long term.

Another role for the nurse is that of counsellor. By promoting the opportunity for the patient to express himself, she can help him to gain a greater understanding of who he is and what he wants in life. As a result, the patient promotes review of his life experiences, and thereby begins to find a basis from which he can grow towards a healthier lifestyle. Peplau sees that patients can use nurses in a way that helps them meet personal needs. The nurse can channel the relationship in such a way as to maximise the opportunities for the patient to do that.

(Nursing roles are discussed further in Chapter 3.)

SUMMARY

Peplau sees the main work role of nurses and their various sub-roles as being important in providing the patient with the best possible opportunities to enhance his life, or to cope with disability or a peaceful death.

Peplau's model is conceptualised in terms of the importance of what goes on within the nurse–patient relationship. It is of major importance for patients to learn about themselves, using their abilities to express themselves fully and freely to a nurse and so maximise their chances of further personal development while moving from illness to health. Peplau also sees nursing as a growing experience for nurses, who learn by observing and studying their patients' interactions with them.

The uniqueness of nursing requires a nurse to exercise many skills; these must be thought about when the nurse is coping with the complexity of interactions with a patient. In this sense nursing is a maturing force which requires understanding of significant therapeutic interpersonal processes.

Health is seen as a symbolic term denoting a forward movement of personality that enables a person to live productively within society. Peplau describes health as a dynamic quality, one which allows the person to feel well and to strive to maintain optimum well-being during his lifetime. She considers that nurses have an important role in being health promoters and educators, as well as having other roles when caring for someone who is ill.

Figure 1.2 Influences on nursing care, as identified by Peplau

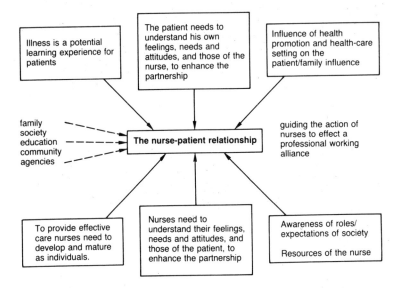

Illness is a potential learning experience for patients

The patient needs to understand his own feelings, needs and attitudes, and those of the nurse, to enhance the partnership

Influence of health promotion and health-care setting on the patient/family influence

family
society
education
community
agencies

The nurse-patient relationship

guiding the action of nurses to effect a professional working alliance

To provide effective care nurses need to develop and mature as individuals.

Nurses need to understand their feelings, needs and attitudes, and those of the patient, to enhance the partnership

Awareness of roles/ expectations of society

Resources of the nurse

CHAPTER TWO

Phases in interpersonal relationships

THE NURSE–PATIENT RELATIONSHIP

The relationship developed between a nurse and a patient is vital to the process of nursing. Making an effective relationship is a dynamic skill which involves not only a thorough understanding of nursing knowledge and skill, but also the confidence to work through difficult issues with patients. Peplau claims that nurse–patient relationships at their best go through four definable phases: *orientation, identification, exploitation,* and *resolution.* Each phase has particular uses and characteristics. While each phase can be discretely described, in practice the four phases also tend to overlap, and earlier phases may be repeated as dictated by changes in the patient's needs. Nurses who are observant and aware of the current phase of the nurse–patient relationship tend to be more effective than nurses who are unaware of this. Peplau sees the potential for a patient to gain a greater insight into his condition using these phases of nursing care.

PHASES IN THE NURSE–PATIENT RELATIONSHIP

Phase of orientation

When a patient becomes ill, either as an emergency or over a longer period of time, the nurse has to help him to become orientated to a totally unfamiliar situation of being in hospital, or to the more familiar one of making his home a 'personal infirmary' while he strives to get better again. In both situations, the nurse has to be empathetic to the needs of the patient, which include becoming orientated to his situation, to new people and to his ill health.

The patient will nearly always be anxious and will forget some of the information given to him. In the orientation phase, therefore, repetition of facts, names and procedures is necessary. Nurses and other professionals providing care need to remind the patient who they are, to explain the purpose of procedures in language the patient can understand, and to explain the work the patient will have to do in order to regain health.

The patient who does not totally understand his condition will need space and time in his orientation; his anxiety will be particularly high in unfamiliar situations. Being wrenched from one's normal activities of working and living at home as a healthy member of the family is traumatic, so the nurse must realise that the phase of orientation is an important one for the patient. If these needs are taken into account, the patient becomes better informed about his condition and can then assess his situation more proficiently. He needs to be able to ask questions; these provide him with information and a greater insight into his situation. As a result the nurse gives him some degree of control in what is often a difficult problem. Orientation is about strangers meeting and coming together: it sets the scene in which the nurse–patient relationship can grow. As Peplau states in her original work, the nurse and patient learn to work in a co-operative manner to resolve difficulties (Peplau 1952).

Phase of identification

Whereas the patient uses the phase of orientation to make a global assessment of what is happening to him, and who in the environment can be relied upon for help, the phase of identification begins when the patient becomes clearer in his mind about his problem. This phase involves the patient identifying with the nurses whom he has experienced as useful to him; he places trust in the staff who do things that they say they will do, and who keep their promises. Patients identify with nurses who are open and honest in their approach and who provide information for them. The problem-solving ability of the patient grows as a result.

In this phase, the nurse–patient relationship can take different directions: the patient can become more involved in his care and enhance the relationship along productive lines; he can avoid involvement, which makes the nurse and patient reflect on their initial contact with each other and the possible associated anxiety; or he can become passive and let the nurse do everything for him. The direction a patient takes will depend on his previous experiences of being nursed, his present condition and the relationship he has established with this nurse. A patient may start by being rather passive but, as he identifies things, become more involved in his care. It follows that the nurse should be looking for patterns of behaviour change: these can give her a clear understanding of what the patient is thinking and feeling.

Phase of exploitation

As the informed patient gains a clearer picture of his situation he starts to identify his needs. The phase of exploitation is characterised by the patient making full use of the resources available around him: the people and the environment. The nurse–patient relationship is the centrepiece, the chief way in which the patient uses his situation and the health professional for his benefit. He seeks more information about his health problem; he checks out the resources around him to see whether they will meet his immediate and long-term goals of health-directed behaviour; he discusses things with other patients to see whether he is gaining the right information. The concept of the patient being in partial control is important here – as he considers his situation his dependency on the nurse is readjusted. The relationship is at a meaningful, productive and potentially informative level in this phase; the planning and implementation of care can be a co-operative process.

The phase of exploitation can be seen as a phase of working through issues for the nurse and the patient, and is seen as a necessary step to take in order to reach the final phase in the relationship. Peplau discusses the point about 'growth cues' being recognised by nurses (Peplau 1952). This dynamic situation involves a change in the nurse–patient relationship from one of dependency (like that of a child to a parent) to one where both the nurse and the patient begin to function in an adult way, identifying and exploiting areas of independence and areas of interdependence. Such behaviour is seen in all the phases, but particularly in exploitation and the final phase, resolution. Patient compliance with or resistance to nursing care is also dictated by the parent–child, adult–adult relationship. Nurses who see the change in behaviour are able to adapt to the striving for independence. Resistance is encountered if the patient fails to benefit from his efforts to become healthy again or if he becomes a 'difficult child' as the relationship fails to grow. The nurse, too, must feel able to deal with problems that inevitably arise in the progress from dependence to independence.

Phase of resolution

Peplau sees the phase of resolution as a 'freeing process', one where the patient begins to take steps to prepare to leave hospital or to live a healthy life at home. Unlike social relationships the nurse–patient relationship is a service-orientated and temporary one: it ends when the work with that patient has been accomplished, or when the care has been passed on to someone else. The termination of care needs to be planned, the patient needs to be prepared for his next situation. It should not be an abrupt termination.

For many nurses, the phase of resolution is the most difficult, as the process of letting go is focused upon. This focus is important because the relationship is one where growth and development take place. The nurse's role in providing the supportive framework in which the patient can free himself must not be underestimated. The type of illness, the age of the patient, the age of the nurse, the length of stay in hospital and the maturity of the nurse and the patient are factors that influence the freeing process. The sense of losing the relationship is countered by the sense of regaining health. It is essential for the nurse to nurture the patient without interfering with the patient's desire to get better.

Moving from one phase to another

There are no hard and fast rules to indicate when a patient moves from one phase to another. Peplau's model should be seen as one in which each phase has defined tasks and roles for the nurse if the relationship is to have few difficulties and problems.

What tells a nurse which phase she is in? The cues mentioned by Peplau regarding growth are indications, helping the nurse see how the relationship with the patient is growing. The characteristics of growth are many, but the work by Knowles (1973) on dimensions of maturation, which indicate the directions of growth, is particularly helpful.

Knowles developed a list of characteristics that produce a clear idea of the concept of growth. The main dimensions listed are these:

- passive–active
- subjective–objective

13

- few abilities–many abilities
- superficial concerns–deep concerns
- ignorance–enlightenment
- dependence–autonomy
- few responsibilities–many responsibilities
- focus of particulars–focus of principles
- impulsiveness–rationality
- narrow interests–broad interests

These dimensions can be applied to the development of a mature nurse–patient relationship. As the patient moves forward with the nurse in growing and developing, the characteristics of maturation change in their focus. For example, as the phase of orientation moves towards the identification/exploitation phases a nurse might see a change in the level of dependency and the emergence of rational behaviour. As a result of experiencing these changes, the patient would move forward by attempting to understand and control his environment and his illness. The nurse would then adapt to the dynamic situation by altering or modifying roles, and in doing so assist the patient to satisfy his needs.

THE IMPORTANCE OF EFFECTIVE COMMUNICATION

The skills of communication, like any other skills, require practice. It is dangerous to assume that communication skills are automatically part of a nurse's repertoire, especially at the level required in a therapeutic relationship.

The following points of communication should be considered as essential requirements for an effective dialogue with a patient.

Listening skills

There is a difference between hearing someone and really listening to them. Listening – especially selfless, one-way, acute listening to a patient, by a nurse – is probably the single most important communication skill for a nurse to master as the basis for a productive relationship with a patient. Listening allows respect to develop, it manifests the interest of the nurse in what the patient is saying, and it provides data essential for the nurse's understanding of what the patient is experiencing. Such attentive listening, however, is a very tiring activity, and sometimes involves tremendous concentration when interacting. It is also something that patients can sense; even the most disturbed person can feel whether a nurse is really listening or not.

Language skills

Coupled with listening is the skill of using language that the patient understands. The use of jargon or complicated words only reduces the speed and quality of an interaction. Where a patient is admitted as an emergency, the process of developing an early trusting link with the person is vital. Yet the chances of this happening will depend on the language skills employed. Using the two skills together, listening and language skills, a nurse becomes a powerful and effective individual. By being effective, the relationship potential is enhanced considerably.

Questioning skills

In the initial relationship, the nurse often has to take the lead in initiating conversation, but once the relationship is established the patient often becomes more involved. As part of the portfolio of skills needed the nurse will have to be able sensitively to assess the patient. The skill of choosing suitable questions will depend on recognising what the nurse needs to know.

In a model of care such as Peplau's the interpersonal skills are expected to be of a high quality, essentially because of the dialogue that goes on between the patient and the nurse. Various forms of questions can be used, and like the other communication skills questioning needs practice. Four types of questions are used most frequently in establishing and promoting the relationship.

Open questions

The aim of this type of question is to encourage the patient to respond with more than a 'Yes' or 'No' answer; they invite the patient to describe what he has noticed about his dilemma. Examples of this form of questioning could be:

- 'What are your present difficulties?'
- 'How long have you been feeling like this?'
- 'So what are your immediate problems?'

Formulating open questions can be hard work, but the potential rewards are much greater than using closed questioning; although the latter is easier to think about it is much less informative.

Linking and clarifying questions

These questions do what they say: link and clarify. An open question can be used initially and the answers given used as the basis of linking and clarifying questions. Examples of these types of questions are:

- 'Could you expand on that point a little more?'
- 'So are you saying that John is the person you are finding hard to get on with?'
- 'Is that the thing you are finding worst of all?'

Extending questions

Like the linking and clarifying questions, extending questions encourage the patient to probe more deeply into a situation. They are useful in a conversation when open questions have been used initially. Examples of this type of question could be:

- 'Are you saying that you expected to be discharged from hospital today?'
- 'Could you say some more on how you behaved when you had visitors last night?'

Extending questions could easily be seen as clarifying questions – this depends on the discussion going on. The important point is that whenever you want more information, the extension of an original question, in order to make more sense out of a situation, is in itself clarifying.

Hypothetical questions

These are helpful in allowing the nurse to visualise how a person may behave or react in future situations. The hypothetical questions give the nurse an idea of what the patient believes might happen and provides some insight into attitudes that have formed in the patient's mind. Examples of this type of question might be:

- 'So what do you think you might do next time this happens?'
- 'So how do you feel you will react when you see Mary again?'
- 'How is this condition going to affect you in the future?'

16

An example

Below is a short dialogue between a nurse and a patient.

Nurse Smith is talking with Mr Brown, who has been in hospital suffering from a ruptured appendix and who has had emergency surgery. He is four days post-operative following appendicectomy. Although the surgery has been successful, Mr Brown has had problems with pain from the wound and is reluctant to move. He has been drinking fluids, but is frightened to eat because he has only had one small bowel action and is feeling full of wind. Although he has been given analgesics and medication to encourage a bowel action, he is anxious generally about being in hospital. Nurse Smith is on duty and seeing Mr Brown. She last saw him yesterday morning.

NURSE SMITH: Hello Mr Brown, how have you been getting along since yesterday? *Open question.*

MR BROWN: Not very well. I feel so bloated with all this wind and my wound is still painful.

NURSE SMITH: So let me check this out a bit more with you.... Have you passed any wind at all? *Linking question.*

MR BROWN: Yes, a little, but I feel there is still a lot to come out.

NURSE SMITH: Have you opened your bowels since yesterday? *Clarifying question.*

MR BROWN: No, but I am sure if I did I'd feel much better.

NURSE SMITH: Do you feel that all this wind is stopping you moving about? *Extending question.*

MR BROWN: Yes, I think so.

NURSE SMITH: Is your wound also stopping you moving? *Linking question.*

MR BROWN: Yes, that's what's worrying me most of all.

NURSE SMITH: So if we can keep your pain under control and sort out the problems with your bowels do you feel you will be able to cope better? *Hypothetical question.*

MR BROWN: Yes and no, I am sure it will help to some extent.

NURSE SMITH: So what else is worrying you? *Clarifying question.*

MR BROWN: Well, I'm not happy about being here, it's been a shock. Last week I was working and I felt fit and happy, and now look at me.

NURSE SMITH: So how long do you think it will take you to get over all this? *Extending question.*

MR BROWN: I think it will take a long time, probably weeks.

This conversation could have taken a number of directions, depending on the questions asked: the questions actually asked here are just one example of using questions to obtain useful information.

Another skill is in the use of silence – sometimes it is better to listen and not speak. Silence can be used to encourage a patient to speak more about what is troubling him. This is an advanced skill; it is sometimes difficult to feel comfortable with silence, to know when to speak and when to remain silent. Yet a nurse needs to be able to cope with silence from a patient, and become used to remaining silent herself.

Peplau's model encourages the development of interpersonal skills and these depend very much on the verbal and non-verbal communication skills identified in this chapter.

SUMMARY

To be skilled in helping people who are ill – to help them to achieve the most favourable outcomes given the circumstances of their situations – a nurse needs to have good skills of communication. In the context of the nursing process, it is essential that the skills of listening and questioning are well practised. The nurse can then enhance the relationship with the patient in a mature and meaningful way. Using a psychodynamic model, Peplau's phases in the interaction can be seen as a process of relationship-building, from the initial trust at the phase of orientation to the exploring of issues with the patient in the phase of identification; a deeper understanding of the patient's needs in the phase of exploitation leads finally to some plan of long-term care with the patient in the phase of resolution.

CHAPTER THREE

Nursing roles

A nurse's relationship with a patient has to be dynamic and flexible: the professional contact with a patient changes all the time. Some of these changes are brought about by the nurse, some by others and some by the person being cared for. Nursing roles within nurse–patient relationships influence the outcomes for patients. Nurses need to have the self-confidence to use roles with patients and to use their professional interpersonal skills to allow the relationships to mature.

Peplau's model recognises that roles are important in developing professional relationships that are dynamic and changing. A role can be described as a set of norms that a person can use in a variety of situations. For nurses the work role and its various sub-roles have to be learned, each one having a different complexity; some are acquired more easily than others. Yet the role of the nurse cannot be considered in isolation, as patient roles and nurse roles interact. Nurses have certain ideas about what the ideal patient roles should be. Such stereotyped perceptions – such as that a patient should ideally be sociable, appreciative, telling the nurse what she wants to hear, and showing certain expected clinical signs associated with the ill health as diagnosed – affect how the nurses behave with the patient. The influence of the perceived roles that nurses expect of patients has been well documented (Stockwell 1972; Johnston 1976), and how patients are talked to has also been explored (Altschul 1972; Anderson 1973; Moult, Melia and Pembury 1978; Faulkner 1979; Breakwell 1987).

The actual problems that nurses have in interacting with patients, coupled with the effect of having a social system and an environment that encourages the nurses to operate in a supportive way, affects the ideal role of the patient being a learner. The professional relationship has the objective of enabling the patient and the nurse to come together and work in a co-operative and mature way. Peplau's developmental model appreciates this approach to care.

NURSING AS A LEARNING EXPERIENCE

Nurses are in a unique position to gain the patient's co-operation and understanding. The potential for the nurse to have a deep professional relationship with a patient is greater than for other professional groups. This potential also means that it is the nurse's responsibility not to abuse or misuse the relationship, for instance to meet her own ego needs. The quality of the interaction is made unique because of the roles that nurses have and the contact time with the patient. If for example a patient is given bad news, there is a high probability that the grieving process will be explored with nurses. The relationship built up between them provides the necessary medium for a dialogue to take place. This is not to say that meaningful relationships with other professional groups do not occur – they do – but the quality of the relationship may be different.

In Peplau's model of care, the consideration of roles is essential as the nurse needs to know how the patient may use them so that his needs can be accommodated (Peplau 1988). Roles in nursing imply a recognition of honesty, of being able to be oneself. As roles are used or adapted the nurse and the patient learn from each other, they learn to accept parameters and boundaries which provide a framework in which to practise. The nurse must consider the long-term consequences for the patient of the roles she takes. By using nursing roles effectively, the patients are encouraged to participate in their own care, to help formulate care plans and solve problems. It is through the phases of interaction that a nurse can identify how dependent a patient is likely to be, and this helps the nurse to predetermine the support that will be needed at various stages of the relationship.

When people are ill, they dispense with some of their social roles: the sick person is much likelier to accept that he needs help. A person's dependency on a nurse and other professional groups is affected by the severity of the ill health, the perceived severity of the illness and the social background of the patient. All these factors also influence a person's ability to manage pain, discomfort and disability. As nurses learn about nursing roles, they have to consider their feelings towards a patient. Nurses may, for example, employ a 'blanket approach' to roles that they have – every patient should be cared for in the same way, with the same emotional detachment; they may feel that personal details of a patient should not influence their feelings and therefore their behaviour. This type of thinking has to be balanced against principles of individual patient care, of looking at each person as a whole and in a personal way.

A nurse–patient relationship can be described as therapeutic if the patient can make a relationship that means he can learn and benefit from that interaction. This, of course, is also true for the nurse.

POSSIBLE ROLES FOR THE NURSE

The nurse as stranger

The 'coming together' process in a professional relationship heralds its beginning. Each nurse–patient relationship is different and Peplau sees the individual approach to care for people as essential if the interaction is to grow in a direction of maturity and co-operative alliance. Strangers must not be labelled or stereotyped; each patient will have a different perception of how he should be treated. In Peplau's view nurses need to offer basic respect for patients, as for any stranger, with the precondition that, unless otherwise proved, the stranger-patient is someone who is intellectually and emotionally capable of understanding what is happening to him.

In practice it is very easy to influence or destroy the potentially positive relationship with an ill person if nurses label people and allocate them into categories for their own psychological convenience. The feelings generated from such labelling or stereotyping outweigh the more productive rational thinking of professional relationships in dealing with people as individuals. Take the example of two patients, admitted to the same ward at a similar time. Patient A is a stranger to the nurses, admitted as an emergency with pneumonia as a complication to AIDS. Patient B is also a stranger, admitted as an emergency with a myocardial infarction. Do the nurses stereotype these patients at all? Perhaps one nurse believes that all AIDS patients deserve what they get, whereas another accepts that some patients with AIDS are innocent victims. Is the care given by these nurses to patient A going to be very different? It is likely that it will be. A comparable difference might occur with patient B: one nurse may say that the patient had been overweight for years and was asking for trouble, whereas another nurse may make no such presumption but treat the patient with respect as she

Figure 3.1 Peplau's phases of interaction and the nursing process

Questions	The nursing process		Peplau's phases of interaction
What are the problems?	Assessment	Collect information; write up a nursing diagnosis	Phase of orientation
What do we need to do?	Planning	Set priorities; write up patient-care goals	Phase of identification
How do we care?	Implementation	Give care	Phase of exploitation
How did it help the patient?	Evaluation	Reassess care; evaluate care	Phase of resolution

The nursing process is cyclical – it has short- and long-term goals of care. There may be more than one cycle of care in each phase of Peplau's model.

Peplau's model is linear – it has a beginning and an end.

would any patient. Who provides the more appropriate, supportive, professional care?

Stereotyping strangers is a dangerous activity, predisposing nurses to think and feel in particular ways, excluding potentially good relationship-building. Peplau's model is useful in getting us to think about individuals and how they need to be cared for in an understanding way.

The nurse as a resource person

In considering the role of the nurse as a resource person, Peplau sees the nurse as someone who 'provides specific answers to questions usually formulated in relation to a larger problem' (Peplau 1988). In practice, it seems that nurses grow into the resource role: they acquire knowledge, skills and attitudes that help them become a useful resource to the patient. They provide information about the hospital or unit, and the various resources in the community. They also provide information on practical matters where the patient might need to develop new skills. To be effective as a resource person the nurse must be effective as a communicator.

The nurse should be aware whether the patient actually needs information, or whether he is asking for support in a disguised form. This is critical; an overload of information, however well-meant, can *increase* his stress. It places the patient in a dilemma – what do I do with this information, what is most important?

The nurse as teacher

The teaching role of the nurse develops alongside the trusting relationship as this builds up over a period of time. As the patient becomes more aware of his situation, the nurse's role of teacher starts to emerge.

The basis of teaching the patient is to work from what the patient knows to what he does not know but needs to know in order to come to terms with his ill health. Assessing the patient's ability to do this is important. Using an experiential approach to teaching, the nurse can generate the learning environments from the experiences discussed with the patient. In this way she can assess the person's capability to be a partner in his care; goals in care can then be agreed and actioned.

Each patient requires teaching in a way that 'tunes in' to his existing knowledge and beliefs. This depends on knowing the

Figure 3.2 The nurse as a resource person

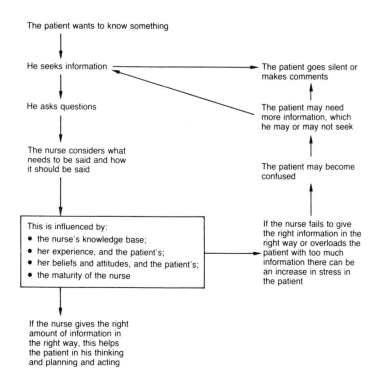

patient well and knowing how the teaching will be received. The nurse as teacher can facilitate the patient in exposing himself to feelings about his ill health. As the nurse teaches the patient, some aspect of his illness becomes clearer to him; there is the potential for a greater understanding of his condition on the one hand, but on the other the growing awareness of what life may be like in the future.

Consider this scenario. Mr Williams is a successful businessman, who in middle age finds that he has maturity onset diabetes. The initial problems he experienced have now been overcome, and providing he maintains his progress he should be able to start work again and lead a full and productive life. Sister Brown, who has been a support to him since he needed help with his diabetes, is teaching him how to recognise signs of hypoglycaemia. At first everything seems to be going well. Mr Williams grasps the essentials of what it can mean to be hypoglycaemic, so from a technical point of view he has understood what can happen to him. Then, as Sister Brown discusses aspects of diabetes with Mr Williams, he appears to stop listening as intently as he did originally. Knowing Mr Williams well, Sister Brown asks him what is troubling him. Thoughtfully he replies, 'I am just beginning to realise what this diabetes is about, it means that my life is going to be different from now on.' The role of teacher can easily alter to the role of counsellor in a situation like this; although this role is discrete it overlaps other roles.

Teaching occurs in all parts of the phases of interaction, but as the phase of resolution is approached, the process of a person freeing himself and taking on responsibility again raises a lot of emotion. In this sense teaching can be emotional as well as instructional; the role of teacher is therefore a potentially delicate one requiring patience and understanding.

The nurse as leader

Peplau explores possible leadership roles in nursing. These can take various guises; realistically, the management and leadership of nurses is influenced by how local health services are run. Management styles in health care affect how nurses manage patients. Policies and procedures that are laid down may transgress the boundaries of professional nursing practice. These factors cannot be ignored; yet at a personal level the nurse and the patient still have the potential to negotiate together in how care should be provided.

An important goal, in Peplau's contention, is that of democratic nursing, where the patient can be permitted and encouraged to organise and to control some or all of his care. To be democratic in leadership, the nurse needs to have confidence in her ability to be flexible and creative. Alternative leadership styles will affect the quality of the role and relationship of a nurse and patient. In situations where there is autocratic leadership, the work with a patient is greatly affected by the local policies and procedures. The leadership style is autocratic and concrete. Nurses in this environment have their professional judgements questioned by the leader, they must justify their reasons for taking a certain approach. This can undermine their confidence in making professional decisions, and increase the pressure to get leadership agreement before setting nursing goals. In a situation where *laissez-faire* leadership prevails, the absence of leadership means that the nurse has little support in proceeding towards goals of caring. Feedback in a positive sense is not forthcoming and the patient can feel threatened by the lack of concrete behaviour from the nurse leader.

For the Peplau model of care to work well the role of a leader needs to be clearly defined in the nurse's mind. This role is often noted and tested by patients as they come to terms with changes in their ill health. A nurse has to be conscious of the potential dependency of a patient on that nurse when certain leadership styles are used.

A useful base-line for nurses meeting new patients is to try to perceive what style of leadership a particular patient will respond to, and whether leadership has to change its form and function as the phases of care develop. The leadership role should be seen as a dynamic one, not a rigid structure with no room for negotiation.

The nurse as counsellor

Peplau sees the role of counsellor as being determined by the purposes lying behind the nurse–patient relationship (Peplau 1988), particularly the promotion of experiences leading to health. Helping a person to become more aware of himself is a skilled process. The art of counselling, to be sensitively accomplished, requires advanced skills in verbal and non-verbal communication. The interpersonal relationship built up in a counselling role can be a very therapeutic one for the patient, where insight into difficulties can be explored. The role of the nurse as counsellor, however, is different from one where a therapist is working with a patient. Counselling by nurses on a one-to-one basis is possible, but it is usually difficult to achieve in practice all the time. Therefore counselling by nurses is often directed toward a particular problem rather than the nurse just 'being there' with a patient.

The counsellor is someone who is willing to sit with someone else to discuss a problem and allow that person to come to some understanding of himself, or to help him draw a conclusion for himself. Not every nurse feels happy about doing this. When a nurse feels insecure in the role of a counsellor there is a tendency to move the conversation to more concrete ground by giving advice. Advice is sometimes all right, but it is not always appropriate; counselling is sometimes all right, but is not always well carried out. The role of counsellor is a difficult one and requires confidence: the nurse needs to be able to see through difficult situations with patients. In practice the nurse usually gets minimal feedback on how things are going so it is hard to visualise how well she is doing in this role.

The education a nurse receives in counselling skills is important because of the potentially difficult aspects of this role. Practice is essential to help the nurse feel confident with the patient. If this is provided, and supported by clinical staff who act as effective mentors for the nurse, counselling becomes a realistic, positive role.

In summary, the following points about counselling are important:

1 Counselling is an advanced skill that requires supervised practice.
2 If the nurse is a good listener, able to reflect back the patient's words as appropriate, counselling is made easier.
3 Counselling involves the exchange of emotion as well as words.
4 It is not easy for the nurse to know when she has reached her maximum level of professional ability.
5 Counselling requires some peer support so that problems can be shared (with the patient's knowledge, because trust is important in establishing a counselling relationship).

The nurse as surrogate

Some patients will use the nurse as a surrogate – a person who functions as a substitute for someone else. When a person is ill, experiences of long ago may become reactivated and the nurse may be seen as a substitute figure. The role of surrogate comes about by patients manipulating situations to diminish their sense of helplessness or powerlessness and to feel more in control of the situation.

The way the nurse responds and behaves affects the surrogate relationship. Suppose, for example, that the nurse reminds the patient of someone else, and the patient actually mentions this: 'You remind me of a girl I once knew.' The nurse can ask, 'In what way am I like this girl?' Having identified the similarity, the nurse can then ask, 'In what way am I different?' This response forces the patient to use his abilities to compare, to see similarities and differences.

For Peplau (1988) the role of surrogate is a potentially useful one, helping the patient to see himself and others as real people, and to allow a deeper, fuller relationship to develop. This role is further emphasised in Peplau's book, where roles are seen as dynamic and ever-changing. As a relationship develops, a maturing of roles also takes place, surrogate roles being particularly powerful. For new nurses, the role of surrogate, like that of counsellor, is a difficult one to handle. Nurses should perhaps consider that being themselves in a professional relationship is the sensible road to take. This allows the patient to experience going through some previous feelings with the present situation. The ultimate movement in surrogate roles is for the patient to move from being childlike to being an adult, making reasonable decisions about his health; the nurse may influence the timing of this transition, and not automatically respond in the surrogate roles offered by the patient. It is important to remember that a surrogate is a substitute and not a replacement: a substitute is by definition 'put in the place of', whereas a replacement 'takes the place of'. Surrogate roles are about substitution.

SUMMARY

A role is a set of norms that a person uses in different situations. Not all roles are used in an interpersonal relationship; each patient is different and so demands different things from a nurse.

Some roles are unique to nurses, simply because nursing is a special kind of caring asking for special skills to be employed so that nurse–patient relationships can flourish. Roles in nursing can be readily identified through the process of care; this is particularly so with the Peplau model, as the phases of interaction serve as a dynamic setting in which roles can be used effectively.

Some roles are taken on more easily than others: the skills and knowledge required vary in complexity. Some roles are possible only if the nurse is mature enough to handle difficult situations. Peer support in some instances is important for success. Nursing sometimes entails handling potentially difficult situations, and providing effective nursing care means learning how to behave with patients in different situations. No two patients are the same.

PART II

Applying the model

It is useful to note that the dependency studies in Part II (Chapters 5–8) do not follow a conventional approach when documenting nursing care. This is to allow the reader to appreciate the versatility of Peplau's model. In Part III of the book there is a discussion on the documentation of nursing care and the reader is invited to consider how efficiently current documentation can accommodate Peplau's phases of care.

CHAPTER FOUR

Peplau's model in practice

Any nursing model where the process of nursing can be used provides an opportunity for the nurse to apply her intellectual and creative skills in actively seeking information about the patient. Nursing care requires that information be obtained from the patient so that accurate goals of care can be identified; the nurse can then make informed decisions, with the patient if possible, on how nursing is to be carried out and evaluated. To do this effectively, a nurse must have practical and social skills to draw upon – nursing involves more than just knowledge. The nurse needs to know how to *behave* with the patient.

As each patient is different, no standard approach is really possible. Nevertheless, any professional who cares for another person requires frameworks in which to practise, so that she can put her generally held beliefs and values to the most appropriate use. With the best will in the world a nurse will not get along with every patient she looks after, and there are bound to be times when problems and difficulties make her feel uncomfortable and even hostile. Nurses, after all, are human beings with feelings of their own.

The nurse's beliefs, values and attitudes come into play with every situation she finds herself in, and become important when she becomes professionally involved with patients. The basis of every successful professional relationship is that nurses should be willing to learn from their patients. Nursing is an interactive process with many facets that contribute to whether the relationship flourishes or fails. The past experiences both of the nurse and of the patient will affect how these two people cope with each other.

A FRAMEWORK FOR PRACTICE

Peplau's model of nursing provides a valuable framework in which nurses can care for their patients in an understanding way. The model recognises that the more the nurse is in touch with what she thinks and feels, the better she is at understanding the reactions of her patients. Nurses knowingly or unknowingly communicate a great deal about themselves to patients, and Peplau tries to recognise this phenomenon in her sequential phases of interpersonal relationships.

Being able to learn from the interaction of a nurse–patient relationship and to recognise difficulties is one of the cornerstones of Peplau's model. But a framework should not be so prescriptive as to cause the nurse to think and behave only in a predictable way. Peplau does suggest in her developmental model that nurse practitioners should expect the unexpected and listen carefully to what the patient has to say. The nurse should learn to follow with one eye those aspects of patient care which she knows well, while keeping the other eye on what she feels she does *not* know about the patient. These two aspects, the knowing and the not knowing, keep a dynamic equilibrium in the care situation.

An experienced nurse does need to make an effort in continuing to recognise that there are things she does not know: she needs to keep an open mind and to be sensitive to new understanding. Peplau's model offers a framework in which the nurse can try to react to each patient's needs, and to be comfortable with each new situation.

Nurses are educated to think about their responses to patients so that they do not respond or behave automatically or inappropriately. However, they tend to develop an attitude to their theoretical beliefs and values which is reflected in how they carry out care. Where elements of similarity exist between past patient care and nursing the patient in the present, the nurse may respond in a routine way. Learning from past experiences is important, but such learning should not become a rigid prescription for practice in the present: effective caring should use past experiences as one basis for nursing practice, without allowing them to dictate a new relationship.

A framework of practice such as Peplau's model should be flexible and durable and help the nurse to think, act and feel; it should be dynamic enough to be used in a variety of clinical care settings. Peplau's model allows the nurse to function comfortably through the interpersonal relationship: it therefore has great potential as a model of action and not just as a theoretical exercise. Nursing in this way should not be a 'trial and error' situation, but one in which the nurse can confidently think, feel, and be intuitive about the patient's needs.

People who are well can think rationally, especially if they are competent, effective, and happy. When people are ill this rationality may blur and they may become emotionally disorganised. This change in the behaviour of a patient provides information which can be part of the developing contract of nursing with that patient.

One use of a framework in practising nursing is in relating the ideas to the care being given. The nurse should ask herself questions about the patient's situation. Should a patient accept certain limits on his lifestyle? Should she help him to challenge negative thinking, given that ultimately only the patient can be the authority on how he thinks or feels? Peplau's model invites the nurse to explore these questions with the patient – to assist the patient to explore, but then to allow him to reach his own conclusions.

CARING WITH FEELING

In the study of nursing models an important question to ask is whether the care for the patient comes with feeling.

Nursing as a science involves the understanding of principles that allow nurses to care for people in a technical way. Procedures are learned in order to provide substance to these principles of care. The *art* of nursing, however, is to recognise that each patient is an individual in his own right. The word 'caring' then takes on extra meaning: caring involves nurses getting to know how patients feel about being ill and how they are coping with it. Nursing involves allowing space for the patients to ventilate what they feel about themselves and to say what they feel about being nursed in the way they are. Feeling positively about being nursed means that the patient, where possible, should be given every opportunity to share his thoughts about what he values.

Nursing is about promoting well-being as well as assisting patients to manage coping with illness, and in this sense Peplau recognises that when people are not well behaviour changes occur which affect relationships. The studies in Chapters 5–8 highlight behaviour change and so emphasise the usefulness of this model of nursing. For now, though, let us consider in general how people may change and feel when they slip into ill health.

The 'ill-health hypothesis' is one which over the years has become more obvious to me. The cycle of events it leads to varies in detail according to the patient's circumstances, age, life experience, and general beliefs in life; to some extent, however, these events seem to occur in everyone, consciously or unconsciously. Our mental state can and does affect our bodily functions, and our physical state of health can affect our mental functioning.

Take the situation of a patient who undergoes surgery. The patient copes physically well with the post-operative phase, but may believe that he could become ill again. This mental state would affect his rate of recovery. Once fully recovered, however, longer-term goals in life take precedence over other shorter-term feelings of not getting better. This I believe is true also of patients who are not going to recover fully. People who have a long-term condition will make slower readjustments to being ill and will at times need greater support by loved ones and by professional carers as they work through feelings of despair. The intensity and duration of an illness will produce a degree of uncertainty and a possible loss of confidence in the patient. Having limited opportunities to share these uncertainties, patients may spiral down into feelings of isolation, of possible guilt, and of helplessness. These feelings cause the person to lose sight of longer-term goals or aspirations (which are much more easily acquired and held when feeling healthy). As a result of this the patient's capacity to cope is reduced, thereby aggravating the problem of trying to cope with ill health. This cyclical problem reinforces further loss of confidence: the patient becomes less able to think and feel positively. Diagrammatically the 'ill-health hypothesis' is shown in Figure 4.1.

Being sensitive about the nursing care she provides, for and with a patient, a nurse can supply the correct environment for developing a professional relationship and in doing so allow support and understanding. At the very least, this caring relationship gives some hope to the patient, an offer of emotional security to help him understand his situation, and the possibility of having some degree of control over his feelings about being unwell. This provides a possible basis for the patient to be involved in his care, and allows the building up of a nursing alliance.

THE NURSING ALLIANCE

Nursing should not be seen in isolation, but as an alliance with other professional groups. Nurses need to form meaningful relationships with patients and colleagues: if they do not, the patients lose out.

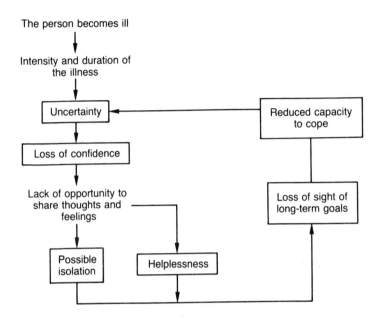

Figure 4.1 The ill-health hypothesis

An alliance with a *patient* implies the nurse providing a form of support. But support comes in various forms, and if effective care is to be provided, then the nurse must be aware of how support can affect the patient's behaviour. There are a number of possible methods of support that nurses can use.

Physical support

Here the nurse measures (sometimes against agreed criteria) what care the patient needs. This forms part of a nursing assessment. If carried out correctly, the patient enjoys a better plan of care, which meets needs and wants realistically. This is where a nurse's skill within a knowledgeable framework becomes important, for without an adequate knowledge base of the science and art of nursing, the alliance with the patient cannot be completely effective. The nurse's relationship with her colleagues must also be effective: if she can communicate and share her findings with other professionals, she will enhance her alliance with the patient as the other professionals, when in contact with the patient, will reinforce the support she is giving.

Emotional support

Here the nurse provides the patient with time and allows a trusting relationship to be built up, promoting the best interests of the patient. The nurse provides an advocacy which enhances the nursing alliance even further. Her emotional support for the patient is also provided through her relationship with the patient's relatives and friends. This supports the patient in knowing that he is loved and wanted.

The nursing alliance is at the heart of proficient nursing care. If the relationship is to be fruitful, emotional support is something that must be achieved early in the care.

Esteem support

Here the nurse indicates to the patient that he is valued as a person in his own right. Esteem involves validating the patient's opinion as important, and learning from the patient as a result of this. By giving value to the patient's opinion a bond is formed that enables trust to develop, so allowing issues of importance for the patient to be explored and discussed.

These three kinds of support – physical, emotional and esteem – allow a stable, more enduring relationship to be formed.

Support for a patient, as viewed by Peplau, must be seen in the context of a social network. The support that is necessary for one patient may not be needed by another. The amount of support will vary according to the patient's condition and general needs. Support cannot be given in isolation, but only in the context of the patient's lifestyle. If needs are correctly identified, the correct amount of physical, emotional and esteem support can be identified and provided.

Nursing in hospital or in the community

The nursing alliance can be understood as relevant in different patient settings. In hospital the patient has little control over his own care, even with the most individual type of nursing care: to some extent, care is taken out of the patient's hands – professionals work within timetables, for example; food is served at particular times of the day. This may be no particular hardship for the patient or the nurse in their relationship, but there is some restriction on the

36

patient's activity. Thus in hospital settings the professionals tend to be in control of the patient.

If the patient can be nursed in his own home, however, he can be much more comfortable. He can be more in control of his care; his relatives can be more involved in providing support and love. The nurse can therefore be an adviser within the patient's social network. Psychologically, this can be very beneficial to the ill person. Health promotion is easier to discuss and effect, and the patient has choices to make in an environment he knows and feels comfortable with.

Peplau's model of nursing is useful in community care. The caring relationship that is needed can be established earlier than in hospital. Early discharge from hospital to home is the growing trend; the planning, implementation and evaluation of nursing care should be transferable, so that what is used in hospital can be used with equal effect at home.

Types of nursing alliance

If we are to try and use a developmental model of nursing, such as Peplau's, we need to understand how an effective alliance can aid recovery of a patient. The way a person is treated psychologically, how he is treated as a human being, will bear directly on his speed of recovery. The more he is seen and respected as a unique individual, the more he will *feel* like an individual. The more personal is the nurse's acceptance of the patient, the less humiliated he feels when intimate procedures are carried out for him.

An ill person has a greater desire to recover if he is respected as human and if he feels that the nurse looking after him actually cares about him. This in turn helps the nurse to feel important and more skilled.

The possible types of alliance with a patient that a nurse can achieve are as follows.

Active–passive alliance

In conjunction with other health professionals the nurse cares for a patient by doing things for him, and the patient accepts this care passively.

When the patient is acutely ill, in pain, unconscious or in some way unable to care for himself without help, this alliance becomes a very functional one. The patient has little say in how he should be treated. In most situations this type of care is useful only for limited periods of time: eventually the patient would become uncomfortable about this authoritarian approach and start to assert some rights. His body, after all, belongs to him and not to the nurse. Yet some patients like to be told what to do and are happy to let decisions be made for them.

In long-term care, one can see the awful consequences of routine care being imposed on people – as, for example, in the population (diminishing, in some countries) of hospitalised patients who have a long-term mental health problem.

Expert–compliant alliance

This is a potentially useful alliance in which the nurse offers expert advice to a patient, which he is expected to agree to. This method of relating is used by a number of other health professionals as well, such as doctors.

When a patient is relatively dependent on a nurse, this alliance can be used frequently; the nurse, for example, may advise the patient not to get out of bed too quickly, but to do so gradually. If the patient has greater control of his physical abilities, however, such a request may be viewed differently by the patient, as though he has a responsibility to comply with the advice and therefore a duty to the nurse.

Co-operative alliance

This is where the nurse and the patient agree with each other on a plan of care, a patient contract. Most patients prefer such sharing of power and responsibility; it gives them some control over what is happening to them. Co-operative alliances are possible also with the doctor, physiotherapist, occupational therapist, dietitian or social worker, and most patients would benefit from this style of care. In the case of a patient having cold orthopaedic surgery, for example, the patient would be able to indicate the most comfortable position to lie in and state what speed he needs to walk at before and after surgery.

In practice this seems to be a relatively unusual alliance, which is a shame as the effect of the care alliance can influence the patient's feelings of progress more profoundly than the personal style of the professional nurse.

In Peplau's model it is the co-operative alliance that is explicitly sought: this seeks to minimise what some patients undoubtedly experience – fear of the professional. Research has demonstrated the reality of such fear in some circumstances; evidence of patients fearing respected doctors (Jarvinnaan 1955), for example, showed that those waiting for a doctor's round in coronary care units were most likely to have relapses in their condition about ten minutes before the round was due to commence. Stress in patients in hospital environments is something that must be accepted as a potential problem in health care. A good alliance, one where the patient is respected and valued, may be a powerful contributor to good recovery.

SUMMARY

The application of a nursing model like that of Peplau requires the nurse to consider her role in relation to the patient. The framework for practice, coupled with the nursing alliance, invites the nurse to use her skills of communication in harmony with her skills of nursing, and to remember that the patient is at the receiving end of all this skill.

Nursing is difficult enough to practise in itself, without the additional pressure of applying an irrelevant nursing model. Peplau's model is very relevant: as a developmental model, it encourages the nurse to develop good human relationship skills and thereby to grow in self-esteem. Good psychological as well as physical support for patients makes the experience of illness easier to bear, both for the patients and for the staff. The development of a sound framework for nursing care is a necessary part of a nurse's function, which can help to prevent the negative aspects of ill health from inhibiting the patient's recovery.

In reading Chapters 5–8, the care studies, you are invited to recall the aspects of caring discussed here, and to consider their value and use within the examples given.

QUESTIONS FOR DISCUSSION

1 How important is it to have a framework for practice when caring for a patient?
2 What aspects of the nurse–patient relationship should always be thought about when planning care?
3 Which nursing alliance do you practise most commonly?
4 How difficult is it, or would it be, to use a co-operative alliance with the patients you nurse?

5 Do you think that the 'ill-health hypothesis' is in reality a problem? If so, is it difficult to prevent?

CHAPTER FIVE

Care study: the young patient

This chapter considers the use of Peplau's model in relation to a young person who has asthma. This dependency study shows Peplau's model providing a framework for practice.

DAVID JOHNSON

David is 4½ years old, the only child of Mr and Mrs Johnson. Since he was born he has always been a sickly, chesty child, and the family decided to move away from the smoky atmosphere of the city and out into the country.

Mr and Mrs Johnson found a reasonably priced pair of cottages which Mr Johnson was going to convert into one larger cottage. During these alterations, however, David became ill again. He started to cough and wheeze and Mrs Johnson had to sit up with him all night, as she had done so many times before when his colds had gone to his chest. By the morning, she was very worried; David was looking grey, his skin was clammy, his nostrils were pinched and flaring, and the skin over his chest was sucking in each time he drew breath. Mrs Johnson could see that David's heart was beating much faster than usual against his chest; he was very restless and was not comforted by her cuddles. She called her new general practitioner who visited immediately and called for an ambulance to take David to the hospital.

David was admitted to the children's ward of the local hospital where he and Mrs Johnson were greeted by the person in charge, Nurse Price. Mr Johnson arrived five minutes later, having followed the ambulance in his car. David was more rested now, and was being given oxygen by mask; an intravenous infusion was in progress. Once David was tucked up in bed, Mr and Mrs Johnson were given

41

cups of tea and Nurse Price invited Mrs Johnson to tell her about David.

'As a baby, every cold David had went straight to his chest. Our doctor called it wheezy bronchitis and said David would grow out of it. As he got older, he used to cough a lot at night, and the doctor gave me some cough stuff. He was a bit better then and only got really wheezy when he had a cold.

'It was worse in the winter, and sometimes I would be up with him for two or three nights before it went. The doctor gave him some antibiotics when it was that bad. It seemed that everyone in the city had colds most of the time during winter, so we thought that if we bought a place further out in the country it would be better for David.

'We found this lovely pair of cottages which his Dad was keen to do up, to make one nice roomy cottage out of the pair. David started to cough and wheeze yesterday but he had no sign of a cold and I couldn't understand why he was coughing. He got much worse in the night – worse than I'd ever seen him before and by this morning I was really worried. I thought he was doing to die.' At this point Mrs Johnson started to cry.

PHASES OF THE NURSE–PATIENT RELATIONSHIP

Phase of orientation

The dynamic of establishing contact

Nurse Price realises that David is ill and will require careful handling and treatment in the next few hours; because he looks so ill, his mother and father will need a lot of support in order to feel in some control again. The fact that Mrs Johnson cried after relating the circumstances prior to David's admission suggests to Nurse Price that Mrs Johnson may have several anxieties. She is also conscious that Mr Johnson has heard what his wife has said: he too is part of this scenario.

Nurse Price makes some observations about David.

Observations

1 David requires oxygen, but possibly only for a short period of time.
2 He needs medication by intravenous infusion (aminophylline and hydrocortisone).
3 He requires a nebuliser every 2–4 hours (salbutamol).
4 He requires careful observation, especially when having aminophylline (because of possible toxicity).
5 He needs to drink frequently, as he will have a dry mouth because of his increased respiratory rate.
6 He will get anxious and restless if he becomes at all anoxic.
7 He is likely to be frightened because he hadn't experienced this degree of bronchospasm before.
8 He will need his parents near him, especially his mother, to provide some reassurance and comfort.
9 He will not want to do much, but will probably be content with listening to a story or watching television.
10 He will probably not feel like eating, but plenty of fluids should be offered.

She also makes observations on Mr and Mrs Johnson:

Observations

1 They need some time to be understood. They need time to talk about David's condition and to build up a relationship with the ward staff and medical and paramedical groups.
2 Mrs Johnson is upset because of her fear of David dying, but also possibly because David's attack was an unexpected setback with his health. She may also feel guilty about moving David into the country, only to find him having one of the worst bouts of illness that she has ever seen him have.

Nurse Price realises that the dynamics of establishing contact with David and his parents are going to be crucial. In summary she has therefore observed the following:

Subjective observations	Objective observations and care
1 David and his parents are going to be frightened: (a) because of the fear of death; (b) because of the strange environment they are in; (c) because they do not know what is happening and what the likely outcome may be. 2 David and his parents will need to have things explained to them carefully in order to get their co-operation. 3 Mr and Mrs Johnson will need to feel in control of the situation as much as possible, and to accept that some support from the professional staff is needed for David.	1 David needs oxygen therapy until the other medication takes effect. 2 David needs to have an intravenous infusion maintained and needs to have a nebuliser every 2–4 hours. 3 Pulse and respiration rate need to be taken and recorded every hour. 4 David requires a regular amount of fluid orally. 5 David needs observing for signs of anoxia. 6 David needs the presence of his parents initially to provide some reassurance in this early part of his care. 7 David and his parents need to have a listening nurse in order for them to cope with their present circumstances.

Nurse Price plans to work towards the following outcomes of care:

1 To ensure that the parents, especially Mrs Johnson, are able to express how they feel about David's condition, and to allow as much time as possible to enable Mrs Johnson in particular to make a relationship with the ward staff.
2 To encourage Mr and Mrs Johnson to continue caring for David while he is in hospital.
3 To work with David and his parents so that a trusting relationship can be built up between them and the staff.

4 To work with Mrs Johnson in particular, to lessen her level of anxiety and to support her so that she can become involved with David's care.

The aim behind this plan is for Nurse Price to help build a consistent supportive network for David and his parents and as a result to allow them to feel as comfortable as possible in the hospital environment. She also seeks to keep Mr and Mrs Johnson's anxiety level as low as possible so that they will be less frightened about David's technical care and will be able to give David the reassurance he needs while he is in the early stages of his treatment. Nurse Price expects that when the parents see David improving the trusting relationship will be built up further between her and the parents and between her and David. In addition, Nurse Price hopes that the doctor's explanation to his parents of David's condition will be of major importance in establishing a trusting relationship. The other members of the nursing staff will be informed of David's admission at a convenient time, and Nurse Price will be looking for the aims of orientation she has outlined to be supported consistently by those caring for David.

As the hospital is some way away from where they live, Mr and Mrs Johnson are offered accommodation overnight. Mrs Johnson elects to stay at the hospital, but Mr Johnson is due at work the following day and goes home.

Over the next twenty-four hours, David improves quite well; his intravenous medication is gradually reducing and he is having nebuliser treatment four-hourly. He continues to drink well, but refuses to eat.

Phase of identification

The dynamic of deepening the relationship

David has been in hospital for twenty-four hours. He seems more settled and the medication has been working well. The doctor has spoken to Mrs Johnson about David's condition, explaining that he has had an asthma attack. Mrs Johnson passes on this information to Mr Johnson when he visits David. Following her initial plan based on her preliminary observations, Nurse Price assesses David's progress:

Subjective observations	Objective observations
1 David seems less anxious and is beginning to enquire about his surroundings.	1 David seems to be responding to treatment.
2 He seems settled in hospital, and shows no signs of being frightened by the nurses or medical staff.	2 His observations (pulse, respiration) indicate that his asthma attack is subsiding.
3 He seems to be forming a firm relationship with Nurse Young.	3 He is communicating with his mother.
	4 He does not like the infusion being in his arm.
	5 He is looking around at some of the other children in the ward.

Nurse Price discusses her observations at a ward staff meeting. The doctor feels that if everything continues to go well the infusion in David's arm can be removed the next day.

Nurse Price wants to develop the phase of identification and get Mrs Johnson to get more involved in David's care. In summary, she wants:

1 To ensure that the initial relationship built up between David, his parents and the professional staff is deepened and made more productive: any questions can then be answered in a more meaningful way.
2 To encourage David to become more independent and mobile.

During the next thirty-six hours, Nurse Price and Nurse Young spend time with both David and Mrs Johnson. They check to see whether Mrs Johnson feels more confident about David's progress and whether she feels able to talk openly about her feelings about David's condition. They check the relationship between David and his mother and father and how dependent he is physically and psychologically on his parents and the members of staff. The infusion in David's arm is removed and he is put on to oral steroids. His nebuliser is continued four-hourly. David is sleeping fairly well, and when awake is eating a little more and drinking well. He is now eager and able to explore his environment.

Phase of exploitation

The dynamic of being flexible

Nurse Price notes the following:

Subjective observations	Objective observations
1 David seems happier than previously.	1 David is coping with his medication and nebuliser.
2 He has formed a strong bond with Nurse Young.	2 There are no abnormal readings for his pulse or respiration.
3 Mrs Johnson appears to be in control of herself and is able to cope with David and Mr Johnson.	3 He wants to get up and walk around and explore.

Nurse Price knows that David will want to play more with other children and will want more attention from his mother and father when he is alone with them. She realises too that there must be a transfer of care responsibility to David's parents and that this needs to be explored with Mr and Mrs Johnson before David goes home. In summary she wishes to evaluate the feelings of Mr and Mrs Johnson about David being discharged home. In specific terms, she plans:

1 To see how David begins to explore the ward, and how easy it is for him to venture away from his mother and make friends with other children.
2 To see whether David becomes wheezy on becoming more active and whether the nebuliser has any effect in reducing this if so.
3 To assess Mrs Johnson's knowledge about asthma, in particular the possible causes of asthma in David.
4 To transfer more responsibility for David's care to Mr and Mrs Johnson, in preparation for his discharge home.

Nurse Price is conscious that Mr Johnson has been heavily involved with David's care and is anxious not to have a further episode with David needing readmission into hospital. (On the other hand, the relationship developed between the professional staff and

David means that with any future admissions the trust would already be there.)

As part of the process of preparing David for discharge, Nurse Price knows that Mr and Mrs Johnson need to be given practical advice and support, to reduce the chances of David needing readmission. She feels that as the relationship is good between the ward staff and David's parents they will probably welcome such advice and support and that this will reduce the level of anxiety about David being discharged home, even though this anxiety may not actually be discussed.

By the fourth day, David appears to be progressing well. He continues to have oral steroids. The nebuliser is replaced by a salbutamol inhaler and a spacer device, which David learns to use. He will take this home to use in any future attacks. He is quite active and has made friends with some of the other children. Mrs Johnson has another talk with the doctor about David and when he may go home.

Nurse Price discusses with Mr and Mrs Johnson how they will cope in the future and how they can manage any further asthma attacks that David may have. She also discusses how David might cope at school and what information should be given to the teachers. She talks about contacting the local branch of the National Asthma Campaign; this will help Mr and Mrs Johnson come to terms with David's asthma and the contacts should provide a useful support network for them all.

Nurse Price talks about how the inhaler should be used, as David will need to have it available in the future. She also makes arrangements to contact the health visitor who can provide support and health education for the Johnsons.

Phase of resolution

The dynamic of feeling in control

Nurse Price makes some mental notes about Mr and Mrs Johnson's reaction to the information she has given them. If all goes well, it is expected that David will be discharged home the next day, with an appointment to see the paediatrician in 4–6 weeks' time in the children's out-patients clinic at the hospital.

Superficially, David's parents seem to accept the idea of David going home. Nurse Price considers however that it is important to assess how, as parents, they are really feeling about David's condition and how they will cope in the future. She wants to be certain that all the obvious points about David's care are understood and to ascertain whether the relationship with David will be any different for them. She would like to know how Mr and Mrs Johnson will react in the future at the first sign of David getting a cold, and whether they are likely to over-protect him.

She wants to find out how David has felt about being in hospital and whether he is looking forward to going home. Mr and Mrs Johnson need to be warned that once back at home children who have been in hospital may be a little more demanding and seek reassurance for a while. But, as Mrs Johnson has stayed with David, this is likely in this case to be less of a problem.

EVALUATION OF CARE

In David Johnson's case, a useful approach would be to ask how well he coped with being in hospital. The process of interaction with specific members of staff would be useful as an indicator of how settled he may have been while in hospital. Reviewing the process of how the relationship developed between Mr and Mrs Johnson and the staff, and how quickly the trust was built up, would be one evaluative tool.

Another indicator in evaluating the effectiveness of the relationship between parents and staff would be the ability of the staff to begin transferring responsibility to the parents, and of the parents to accept the responsibility without an undue increase in anxiety. This could be outlined as in Figure 5.1.

When one is evaluating the care of a child such as David, there is the added responsibility of considering his parents in that care. The most useful way to provide nursing care to David is *through his parents*, ensuring that they are involved at each stage of management. Evaluation of care can then follow the same route: how well David responds to treatment is reflected in the dynamics of interaction, trust, responsibility and control in the parents. The relationship becomes a triangle of interaction.

In assessing, planning, giving and evaluating care, the triangle of interaction must always remain intact. If one part of it fails, the process of care breaks down. Caring for a young patient, such as David, requires care to be provided in a truly holistic way. Many other people become involved in the care of children; the adequacy of the complex interactions should never be taken for granted.

Figure 5.1 The dynamic of accepting responsibility and retaining control

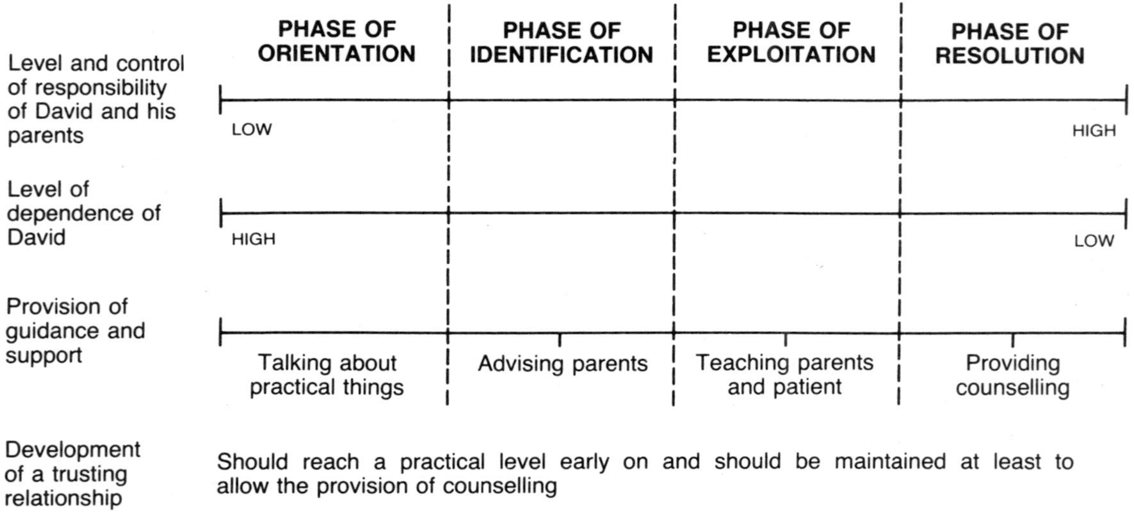

	PHASE OF ORIENTATION	PHASE OF IDENTIFICATION	PHASE OF EXPLOITATION	PHASE OF RESOLUTION
Level and control of responsibility of David and his parents	LOW			HIGH
Level of dependence of David	HIGH			LOW
Provision of guidance and support	Talking about practical things	Advising parents	Teaching parents and patient	Providing counselling
Development of a trusting relationship	Should reach a practical level early on and should be maintained at least to allow the provision of counselling			

The level of control gained will depend upon the corresponding reduction in physical care. This is influenced very heavily by the provision of support for those who require it. The whole dynamic is itself underpinned by the development of the trusting relationship.

Figure 5.2 The triangle of interaction

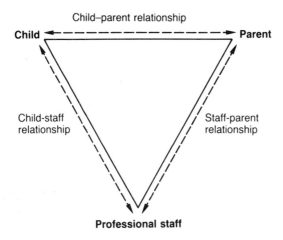

Child–parent relationship

Child ← – – – – – – – – – – → **Parent**

Child-staff
relationship

Staff-parent
relationship

Professional staff

QUESTIONS FOR DISCUSSION

1 In practice, does the Peplau model of care provide a good framework for nursing ill children?
This is useful as a small-group activity followed by a whole-group discussion. Allow at least an hour for this activity.

2 What specific points should you think about when attempting to build up a relationship with a child and his parents?
This is useful for individual work, followed by group discussion. Allow an hour for this question.

3 What anxieties do parents often express when their child is admitted as an emergency? If no anxieties are expressed, what prevents the parents discussing them?
This is useful as a whole-group activity. Allow an hour for this activity.

4 The phase of resolution may have to extend many months past David's discharge from hospital. What are the implications for:
 (a) nurses practising in the community?
 (b) nurses communicating the Johnsons' support needs to community nurse colleagues?
Work individually, then bring your ideas to a small group. Pool your ideas and draw conclusions.
Allow up to 1½ hours for this activity.

51

CHAPTER SIX

Care study: the elderly patient

This chapter considers the use of Peplau's model as a supportive nursing framework when caring for an elderly man who has a confusional state. This dependency study allows us to see how care can be provided to alleviate what is a potentially common occurrence in an elderly person.

MR WILLIAM BROWN

Born in London, William Brown was one of a number of children who lived in some poverty. His father and mother worked hard to keep the family together. When William left school he worked for a building firm, but during the Second World War he was called up and joined the army. During the post-war years William developed his skills as a builder. He married Pearl and they had two children, who eventually grew up and left home. Eventually, at 65 years of age, William retired.

During his working life he had been fit and well, and this continued into his early years of retirement. Pearl now takes up this story and describes what happened to William.

'My husband has always been a strong man physically, never having any serious illnesses, so when he got this cold the other day I was a bit surprised. He went to bed and slept a lot, but instead of getting better, he started to get angry and shouted at me a lot, saying how he thought I was trying to hurt him. He looked so hot, but he wouldn't let me near him.

'I knew he was ill, but I felt so helpless and angry with him because I didn't know what to do. In desperation, I called the doctor and he said that my Bill had a bad chest infection which was causing all the trouble. The doctor said that he was to stay in bed and have lots to drink; he also said he would need something for the infection.

'I had to get to the chemist with the prescription, but I was worried about leaving Bill on his own. Fortunately Mrs Briggs next door was passing, so I asked her if she could get the tablets for me.

'When she got back from the shops, Mrs Briggs came in and had a cup of tea. She could see that I was upset, so she asked me what was the matter; I felt embarrassed but I tried to tell her, but all that came out were tears. I was so worried that Bill was going to die.

'After she went, I gave Bill one of the tablets – it was penicillin, and he took it like a lamb. He slept all night, mumbling from time to time, and he was sweating a lot. The next morning he refused to take the tablet and spat it out saying that I was trying to kill him; he really upset me, he wasn't my Bill any more, he was someone else.

'I phoned the doctor again, and he said he would come later that morning. He said for me not to worry, but what else could I do?

'Then it happened. Bill came down the stairs in his pyjamas and went into the garden to do some digging. He thought it was warm and he tried to take his clothes off – he refused to come inside, swearing at me and telling me to leave him alone. Mrs Briggs saw what was happening and she came and helped me to get Bill inside the house. I felt so awful and ashamed, but I couldn't manage him on my own. Once he was indoors we locked the doors, and tried to calm him down.

'Eventually the doctor arrived and said that Bill needed some treatment in hospital; so he called an ambulance and we took Bill into hospital.'

PHASES OF THE NURSE–PATIENT RELATIONSHIP

Phase of orientation

The dynamics of interaction

Mr Brown is admitted into a Care of the Elderly ward in the local District General Hospital. Sister Fullright is in charge, and after introducing herself to Mr and Mrs Brown she welcomes them into the ward. She enlists the help of Student Nurse French and together they get Mr Brown into bed and settle him down. The initial observations on Mr Brown show that he is pyrexial and unable to communicate properly. Mrs Brown answers most of the questions.

The duty doctor is called and she examines Mr Brown, saying that he has a severe chest infection and will need to be in hospital for a few days. Mrs Brown seems upset at this and asks a lot of questions seeking reassurance that her husband will make a full recovery.

Sister Fullright makes the following observations:

Subjective observations	Objective observations
1 Mr Brown seems confused.	1 Mr Brown is pyrexial and looks ill.
2 His attention span is poor.	2 He has a noisy chest.
3 He seems anxious.	3 He needs things explaining to him several times before he co-operates.
4 Mrs Brown seems frightened of the situation.	

Sister Fullright reflects on the observations she has made. She realises that her role as a stranger might contribute to Mr Brown's confusion and possible non-co-operation. She also reminds herself of the importance of developing a positive relationship early on in the orientation phase (see page 21).

She discusses this role with Student Nurse French, stressing the importance attached in initiating a therapeutic contact with Mr Brown and his wife. She also talks about the role of leader (see page 25) and the need to take the initiative in conversations, to direct the dialogue to meeting Mr Brown's immediate physical and psychological needs. The discussion with Nurse French touches upon the provision of a framework of practical support and guidance for Pearl.

In summary Sister Fullright plans:

1 To ensure that Mr Brown is encouraged to describe what he is experiencing, that he is listened to very carefully, and that his feelings about being in hospital are accepted and understood.
2 To work with Mr Brown so that he can begin to recognise his need for support and accept his dependency on the staff while he is so ill.
3 To work with Mrs Brown to lessen her anxiety and feelings of helplessness and encourage her involvement in Mr Brown's care.
4 To talk to the medical and paramedical staff about her plan to gain their support, understanding and cooperation.

By following this plan Sister Fullright hopes to provide a baseline of consistent behaviour with Mr Brown, and thereby lessen the risk of his regressing. In addition it is her aim to provide a sense of security for him and Mrs Brown, and to demonstrate through her behaviour that Mr Brown is a valued individual. She will note the quality of interaction between them and through this begin to assess how well he is coping with her and the necessary procedures.

As time progresses, William has a chest X-ray and his urine and blood are tested. The doctor is reluctant to sedate him but prescribes a broad-spectrum antibiotic. The nurses wash him, and provide him with a regular mouthwash. He is given a sputum pot and some tissues and shown where these are and how to use them. He has his bowels open, using a commode by the bed, and he is offered a urinal regularly.

Phase of identification

The dynamics of selectivity

Bill has been in the ward for twenty-four hours. Pearl has visited once; she stayed a long time, talking with Bill. He remains pyrexial but he is drinking quite well and taking some light food. Following her initial plan, Sister Fullright assesses what is happening to him.

Subjective observations	Objective observations
1 Bill seems still to be confused at times.	1 He is still pyrexial.
2 He still seems anxious sometimes.	2 He is co-operating quite well with most people.
3 He seems to want to know more about his condition.	3 He is asking some questions.

Sister Fullright discusses these observations with the doctor, with Student Nurse French and with the ward physiotherapist. It seems that Bill is not very pleased to see the physiotherapist. Sister Fullright recognises that he is beginning to organise himself a little more effectively and is showing signs of beginning to relate well with one or two people, but less so with others. She decides to promote the phase of identification by responding to his questions and ensuring that where possible Bill becomes involved with his care. In

55

doing this she hopes to see a change in his behaviour from being a confused, vulnerable person, to one who is achieving independence. In summary, Sister Fullright plans:

1 To develop a trusting relationship to a greater depth than before, to help Bill express his thoughts and feelings more adequately.
2 To get Bill to take some responsibility for his care, and to observe how willing he is to get involved.
3 To help him to understand his illness and why he is behaving as he is with the staff and with Pearl.
4 To see who has his trust and co-operation, and why.

During the next twenty-four hours, Sister Fullright talks with Pearl and assesses how well she is coping. She also discusses with the ward staff, the physiotherapist and the doctor her observations on how Bill is progressing. The antibiotics seem to be taking effect and, combined with the physiotherapy, Bill is coughing productively. The sputum is sent for culture and sensitivity. As the pyrexia is subsiding he appears to be more lucid and co-operative. His relationships with Sister Fullright and Student Nurse French seem particularly good and he likes talking with them. It is agreed that Bill should be mobilised and that an arrangement be made to discuss the care he needs with him and Pearl.

Phase of exploitation

The dynamics of control

Sister Fullright makes the following observations:

Subjective observations	Objective observations
1 Bill seems less confused.	1 His pyrexia is subsiding.
2 He seems less anxious.	2 He is co-operating well.
3 He seems to be more settled.	3 He is asking selective
4 He seems to relate to some	questions.
people well.	4 He is taking some personal
	control over his care.

She anticipates that Bill will soon start to identify what he likes to do and when he likes to do things, and that he will start to check out what he can do on his own, such as have a proper bath, get out of bed, and go to the bathroom to shave. She expects that as time goes on and he gets stronger, goals about going home might be discussed. She knows that the recognition that he has choices is important to him.

In summary, Sister Fullright plans to evaluate the effect of care so far and to assess Bill's ability to take on some form of assisted independence. In particular she plans:

1 To see how Bill's behaviour is changing and whether he accepts some responsibility for his care.
2 To check whether the staff involved in his care are able to let him become more independent, or whether there is a risk of him being overnursed.
3 To see how well the staff, Pearl and Bill are co-operating with each other.
4 To identify potential or actual problems that prevent him from progressing.

She may question how the staff feel about Bill now that he is doing more for himself, and whether the initial work done in building a trusting relationship has paid dividends.

Phase of resolution

The dynamics of independence

The following observations are made about Bill:

Subjective observations	Objective observations
1 He seems lucid.	1 His temperature is normal.
2 He seems in control.	2 He co-operates well.
3 He feels at home.	3 He wants to do things for
4 He is relating well to Pearl.	himself.
5 He is more demanding.	4 He talks well with Pearl.
	5 He wants to talk about going home.

Five days have elapsed since Bill's admission to the ward. He continues to have his antibiotics, and the physiotherapist helps him cough up his sputum. He is X-rayed again and has further blood tests to check his progress.

Bill has been ambulant for two days and although weak is able to wash himself and to shave. His urine is clear and his bowel movements seem regular. He is eating regularly, mainly solid food, and is drinking well.

Sister Fullright considers that Bill is able to take care of himself physically, but recognises that psychologically he has had a shock; he was very frightened about becoming confused and aggressive. She also feels that Pearl may have anxieties about him becoming ill again and is likely to seek support from the staff. She also knows that Bill needs to take on the full responsibilities of life again and that this is a major psychological step.

In summary, Sister Fullright wants to assess the following:

1 Has Bill worked through all the issues surrounding his illness before going home? If so, he will feel more in control when at home.
2 How well will he begin to let go of the relationship that he has with the staff? He needs to be free, to be 'psychologically discharged'.
3 How will his relationship with Pearl compensate for his loss of contact with the ward staff?
4 How well has he adapted to making his own decisions?
5 How well can he accept advice about staying healthy in the future?

Thinking about her role as a resource person and teacher (see page 23), Sister Fullright suggests a time when Bill could be discharged home. She observes his reaction to this suggestion. Aware of her need to communicate effectively and not to overload him with information, she talks through what it would mean to him and Pearl for him to be sent home.

As a group, the three of them discuss Bill's and Pearl's present home circumstances: it is agreed that the community nursing service be advised of Bill's discharge so that they can visit him to see whether he is maintaining his health. In addition, the doctor decides to see Bill as an out-patient and in the meantime to write to his general practitioner about the treatment he has had while in hospital.

The planning of his discharge home involves the role of counsellor as well (see page 26). Sister Fullright and the ward staff provide 'talking and thinking time' for Bill and Pearl. The psychological process of coming to terms with the ending of this professional relationship has to be acknowledged. There is the recognition that Pearl will become the main, consistent support for Bill while he recovers.

EVALUATION OF CARE

The care Bill received and its effect on his recovery need to be evaluated. Psychologically, too, the dynamics of care can also be evaluated: how well is he coping with the thought of going home? When this is suggested, does his behaviour show an increase in dependency or is his reaction one of acceptance and readiness to go home?

The evaluation of the effectiveness of care should also consider the trust present within the nurse–patient relationship. How honest can the staff and Bill be with each other? Is it important to ask Bill whether he feels confident enough to go home, and to check whether he has realistic expectations about his ability to cope with his recovery? What is Bill's apparent level of anxiety? When it is suggested that he go home, does he show signs of being defensive or evasive? Such a response could indicate that there are hidden feelings or issues around for Bill which have not been properly discussed, recognised or resolved.

What are Pearl's feelings about Bill coping at home? Is she ready to assist him? How well has the relationship developed between Pearl and the ward staff?

Above all, the evaluation should consider the level of independence achieved by Bill and Pearl. How quickly did they move to a state of independence?

How fit is Bill psychologically to decide to go home? How well will he take on the responsibility for his own care?

QUESTIONS FOR DISCUSSION

1 How much emphasis should be placed on initiating relationships with elderly confused people? Is it necessary to do this if the person fails to understand what you are saying?
2 As a communication tool, how valuable is the skill of touching in caring for someone who is confused?

EXERCISES

1 Consider three ways that you could communicate with a confused person. Write these down. Think about the advantages and disadvantages for each method you have listed, from your own point of view.

   Which method seems easiest to use, from your point of view?

   Which method do you think would be the easiest for the confused person to use with you?

   How would you evaluate the progress you were making with a confused person through these methods of communication?

   You need to allow about an hour for this exercise.

2 'Peplau's model recognises that roles are important in developing professional relationships that are dynamic and changing' (page 19). Which roles would you consider are used most of all by nurses when nursing a patient like William?

   What are the short- and long-term consequences of these roles? You might wish to re-read Chapter 3 and list your ideas. Working in small groups, check each other's ideas and draw conclusions.

   You should allow about 1½ hours for this activity.

CHAPTER SEVEN

Care study: the patient admitted as an emergency

It takes some time for the psychological effects to hit home when someone is admitted as an emergency. For the patient it involves disbelief, followed by possible anger. It is probable that the person will eventually accept the situation, but some people never fully accept what has happened to them. A person who denies what is happening to him is using a defence mechanism that on one level helps him cope with his immediate problems yet on another level prevents him from equipping himself with the psychological tools he needs to cope with the longer-term implications.

Feeling out of control and vulnerable is extremely unpleasant: it also tends to stoke up the level of anxiety being experienced (this is discussed further in Chapter 9). The behaviour of patients varies. Some are calm about their situation and accept their fate; others ignore it and hope that it will go away; others rationalise, and ask 'Why me?'; yet others are angry and uncooperative with the people who care for them or love them. For the relatives of a patient admitted as an emergency, the fear of having their future lives disrupted can be a major focus of concern. Relatives will often try to put on a brave face, so as to be seen as giving support to the affected person; others may make light of the situation and make superficial jokes or comments to help them cope with what is, in reality, a serious situation. In one sense it seems that relatives have more difficulties to cope with than the patient – although the patient is the one who has been experiencing the emergency and the one who is in pain and discomfort, it is the relatives who have the problem of 'learning how to worry' without causing themselves or the patient undue stress. In practice, it is usually the *types* of questions asked by relatives that give the nurse clues as to how anxious and worried they really are.

In this chapter, we look at a patient admitted as a surgical emergency. The patient will probably show signs of anxiety: the nurse can judge from these how to behave with the patient. A lot of the physical care he will receive will be routine or mechanistic. The following patient dependency study uses Peplau's model applied to the general setting of a surgical unit.

MR THOMAS RICHARDS

'My name is Thomas Richards, Tom to my close friends. I have been asked to tell you about what happened to me recently when I became ill, and how I felt about it.

'Let me begin with a bit of background. I am 60 years old, and a Welshman. Besides being a bank manager, I am a lay preacher in the local Baptist Church. Some Sundays I take a service in a local Chapel, especially at busy periods or when the minister is ill or away.

'I am single, but I have a lot of close friends. I have a brother, who lives two hundred miles away, whom I see twice a year; and a sister who lives in New Zealand, whom I haven't seen for twenty years.

'The other day, it was a Saturday, I started to feel unwell and I had a pain develop in the left side of my groin. It came on all of a sudden. At first the pain wasn't too bad, but it became worse as time went on and I started to feel sick. I remember saying to myself, "Come on, get this under control, you've got a sermon to finish for tomorrow morning." I felt so cross that my body was doing this to me, especially as I had this important service to run the next day.

'But it was no good, I started to vomit, and the pain became unbearable in my groin, especially when I was being sick. I phoned Dr Trenchard, my local GP. He was out on a call, but his wife said he would be home soon and she would give him the message that I needed to see him. I felt so ill and when I knew that I had to wait to see my GP I felt very vulnerable and alone. I wanted to have my brother there and through the pain I rationalised that if I rang him he couldn't do anything for me anyway and it would only cause him to worry.

'I then thought about ringing the ambulance directly and felt angry at myself for not doing that in the first place. Here I was, crawling about being sick waiting for the doctor.

'What seemed to be an eternity passed by; I was vomiting in the toilet and on the carpet and down my clothes. The pain in my groin made me wet my trousers. I thought I was dying. Then the front door bell went, it was the doctor. "Thank God for that," I said to myself and got to the door. Dr Trenchard took one look at me and said, "Good God, Tom, what have you been up to?" I was never so glad to see his face.'

Dr Trenchard could see that Tom had a probable intestinal obstruction due to a strangulated hernia, and he admitted him directly to the surgical unit at the local hospital. By the time Tom arrived it was 1.30 a.m. on the Sunday morning.

The night nurse was Staff Nurse Phillips, who was doing a series of nights as an internal rotation shift. When Tom was admitted, Staff Nurse Phillips introduced herself, then took down information about him and where he lived. She asked him about what had been happening and took his temperature, pulse (rate, rhythm, volume) and respiration (rate, depth, regularity), and also took and recorded his blood pressure. Armed with this information she contacted the surgical registrar who came and examined Tom.

PHASES OF THE NURSE–PATIENT RELATIONSHIP

Phase of orientation

Although for Staff Nurse Phillips the admission of Tom is routine, she is aware that for him it must be very frightening. She notes that he is in a lot of pain and that he has trouble answering her questions. She also notes that physically if nothing is done he is going to get worse than he currently is. The registrar puts up an intravenous infusion and prescribes an analgesic, Pethidine, by injection. He takes some blood samples, and orders a chest and abdominal X-ray. Staff Nurse Phillips makes the following observations:

Observations (assessment)

---

1 Tom is vomiting. He has severe pain in his lower abdomen.
2 He finds it difficult to answer questions (the pain is too severe).
3 He is uncertain what is wrong with him and what will have to be done for him.
4 He has wet trousers on and is embarrassed by this.
5 He is worried about who will take the service at 11.00 a.m. today at the local Baptist Church, as no one knows he is in hospital.
6 He seems unable to grasp what has happened to him.
7 He seems to be co-operating with me as much as possible. He wants me to call him 'Tom'.

Staff Nurse Phillips makes this nursing plan of action, bearing in mind the relevant medical factors:

1 Tom must be given nil by mouth.
2 Test the urine and record the results.
3 Prepare Tom for theatre. The abdomen is too painful to be shaved.
4 Organise X-rays, blood tests and consent, with the registrar. Make sure that Tom has adequate information about what is happening to him (from both nursing and medical staff).
5 Establish an intravenous infusion regime of dextrose and normal saline.
6 Control the pain by analgesia and explanation.
7 Attempt to pass a naso-gastric tube.
8 Make half-hourly observations of blood pressure, pulse, respiration and level of pain.
9 Wash Tom carefully as part of theatre preparation.

Summary of management and administration

Staff Nurse Phillips has prepared Tom for surgery, and has organised with the registrar for blood to be analysed, X-rays to be taken and drugs to be prescribed. The intravenous infusion is established and running using alternate normal saline and dextrose 500 ml, four-hourly. A naso-gastric tube has been passed and his stomach has been aspirated. He has passed urine. No urinary catheter has been inserted. He has not been abdominally shaved. His consent form has been signed and he has had 50 mg of Pethidine to control the pain. He has been allowed nothing by mouth. He is too ill to be weighed.

Staff Nurse Phillips knows that she and Tom are strangers and that Tom is placing a lot of trust in her because he has no other option. She knows that he asked her to call him Tom, and feels that this may be an important part of Tom coming to terms with his situation and accepting help from people whom he doesn't know.

She knows that if Tom fails to understand what is happening to him the level of anxiety he is experiencing will become very high; this would cause his pain to increase, and would be likely to increase his vulnerability to complications. So in simple language she informs Tom of every action being taken with him to deal with his immediate distress. She believes that when someone experiences pain which he does not understand, the pain tends to increase. She knows that

Tom has not been psychologically prepared for surgery and consequently the relationship-building between them is vital to help Tom in the post-operative phase of his care. She is also aware that he is worried about the church service and that he will need to feel reassured that someone can be contacted.

In specific terms, Staff Nurse Phillips notes the following points:

1 Tom needs as much selective information as possible before surgery to help him cope post-operatively; but we mustn't overload him with too much information. He needs to know what is wrong and what may have to be done to put it right. He needs to know what tubes will be in him on return from surgery.
2 Those who care for him can have a reassuring effect. A calm person who is confident in communication has a controlling effect on an anxious patient like Tom.
3 Tom will be dependent on the nursing staff, and the relationship established after surgery will be one where the surrogacy role could arise. Leadership skills – in organising Tom's care – will also be needed until he begins to free himself from this dependent vulnerable state.

The initial relationship with Tom has been built up through contact with Staff Nurse Phillips as she has been preparing him for surgery. It is an important first step in helping him retain some control over his situation.

Tom goes to surgery. He has a laparotomy followed by a reduction and repair of a left strangulated inguinal hernia. No gut resection is required. During surgery, intravenous antibiotics are started; these are prescribed for three days, to be given by bolus injection. His intravenous infusion is continued using a four-hourly regime of dextrose and normal saline. His naso-gastric tube is on free drainage and is to be aspirated hourly following surgery. He is prescribed analgesics by injection and this is to be reviewed twenty-four hours after the operation. Tom's laparotomy wound is sutured using Dexon. There is no drain in the wound. Post-operatively Tom is to receive nil by mouth.

Phase of identification

It is 5.30 a.m. when Tom returns from theatre. Staff Nurse Phillips realises that he has had only a limited opportunity to review his situation since admission four hours earlier. However, she also knows that the time she spent with him helped him clarify his situation to a reasonable extent. She expects that on his first post-operative day Tom will be wanting to know what happened in surgery so that he will be better able to cope with his feelings about being in hospital, the visitors he will have over the next 24–48 hours, and the pain and discomfort following his operation. She knows that relationship-building for Tom, such that he can identify with certain staff and feel that he is supported, will be very important for him; if good relationships are established Tom is much more likely to co-operate with people and to get involved in his care.

The following plan of care was identified:

1 Get Tom to co-operate with deep-breathing exercises and leg movements to avoid deep vein thrombosis and in general to avoid stiffness.
2 Mobilise him later today – walk around the bed, sit in a chair. Co-operate with the physiotherapist.
3 Bed bath today; check skin for bruising or other abnormalities.
4 Offer urinal hourly at first, then as often as Tom wants.
5 Intravenous infusion – four-hourly regime continued as per prescription.
6 Nil by mouth. Provide two-hourly mouth care, nasal care.
7 Aspirate naso-gastric tube hourly, keep on free drainage.
8 Observe pulse, respiration and blood pressure hourly until stable; then four-hourly. Continue four-hourly temperature and wound observation.
9 Continue intravenous antibiotics as prescribed; give analgesics as required.
10 When possible, provide time for Tom to encourage him to express his responses to the hospitalisation experience, and find out how well he is coping. Identify his level of anxiety and how well he has adapted to being in hospital.

By breakfast on Sunday morning, Staff Nurse Phillips has handed over to the day staff and makes a last check on Tom before going home. He is asleep, so she doesn't disturb him. She has handed on to Staff Nurse Jones who reads the surgeon's operation notes and re-checks the care plan that Staff Nurse Phillips has compiled. As the unit is an approved area for general nurse training, Staff Nurse Jones organises an experienced student to care for Tom during the rest of the morning. The ward is busy and the staff nurse is able to see Tom only briefly. She is therefore relying on Student Nurse Anderson to report on Tom's physical and psychological state when required.

Eventually Tom is washed, and after the naso-gastric tube has been aspirated, he is offered analgesia. The intravenous infusion and wound is checked and his observations taken and recorded. He is then mobilised and put in a chair by the bed. The physiotherapist on call checks Tom's chest and shows him the breathing exercises he must do. The doctor comes late in the morning and checks Tom's wound, asking him how he feels. He replies that he feels bloated and in pain but that he will manage. Checking the observation and fluid charts, the doctor smiles and says he will see him again tonight.

Tom passes urine and tries to settle over lunchtime as the other patients are eating food. He knows that he cannot eat yet, but wonders how long the naso-gastric tube is to be kept in place.

Tom now begins to assess his situation. It is 3 p.m. on Sunday afternoon. 'Well, I am in a mess now, aren't I? This tube down my nose is really uncomfortable, it's making the end of my nose sore. This drip in my arm hurts. They told me not to move my arm unnecessarily otherwise the needle might fall out, I wonder what they mean? If it does fall out, will I bleed to death? . . . Don't be silly, of course I won't! . . . How do I know?

'What the heck have they done down below – I know that student nurse told me but I can't remember, and that doctor was in such a hurry I didn't like to ask him. He did smile at me – does that mean everything is OK? Or is that a way of saying it isn't? After all, he said he was coming to see me again tonight.'

Tom is identifying his problems to himself and beginning to consider whom he can communicate with to understand his situation more effectively, and to discuss his needs (the phase of exploitation). The relationships with Student Nurse Anderson and Staff Nurse Jones seem different from that with Staff Nurse Phillips. He is going to co-operate, but the initial relationship with Staff Nurse Phillips seems very special to him, and he hopes that she will be on duty again this evening.

Tom is put back to bed later in the afternoon and he has his first visitor, the minister from the Baptist Church. He reassures Tom that they covered his sermon that morning, but that some of the congregation were worried about him. Tom felt much better when he heard the news from the minister. He could then talk about what had happened to him. The minister said he would come to see him again tomorrow. Tom was asked if he would like his brother to be contacted; he said yes.

By 9 p.m. on Sunday, he was feeling in some pain and was given an injection of Pethidine. Staff Nurse Phillips was on duty again and Tom felt very pleased to see her; she, it seemed to Tom, was also pleased to see him. At 10 p.m. Staff Nurse Phillips was able to spend fifteen minutes with Tom, checking his tubes and his wound and making observations. At 11 p.m. the ward was quiet but fairly busy; Tom couldn't sleep very well. After a while Staff Nurse Phillips noticed that he was awake, and came over and checked everything again. She asked him what sort of a day he had; he talked about the thoughts he had been having that morning, about his anxiety. She listened carefully.

After Tom settled, she noted the following observations:

Observations

1 Physically he is standing up well. Post-operative recovery seems uneventful.
2 All observations are satisfactory (no abnormality).
3 Naso-gastric tube aspirated four-hourly and on free drainage.
4 Intravenous infusion four-hourly, with normal saline and dextrose.
5 Six-hourly intravenous antibiotics, four-hourly analgesia given with effect.
6 Mobilised today. Physiotherapist came – breathing exercises undertaken.
7 Passing urine, bowels not opened, no bowel sounds, no flatus passed.
8 Doctor came this morning; did not come again as he said he would.
9 Tom is anxious still. Had a possible problem relating to the day staff: felt they were too busy to deal with his questions and didn't want to bother them anyway because they had more important things to do.

Staff Nurse Phillips could see that Tom's needs were very great this morning. He was vulnerable and in pain. Physically he had good care, but psychologically he is still coming to terms with being in hospital.

Phase of exploitation (1)

By Monday morning Tom is feeling better in himself, although physically sore. Staff Nurse Phillips asks him what things he would like to do for himself and what help he would require. The aim here is to get him to take some responsibility and to have the opportunity to gain some control over his situation. She is attempting to actively promote the forward movement of Tom's personality from that of dependency to independence; in doing so she is giving him the opportunity to readapt to his adult role. Staff Nurse Phillips has recognised the need for Tom's 'growth' to develop into a more positive and responsible behaviour pattern. Before going off-duty, she discusses with the nurse in charge her objective and subjective observations on Tom, and in particular his need to work through some of the issues in his mind. Student Nurse Anderson is briefed as to Tom's needs, particularly the need to be well informed and in control.

The registrar makes a ward round and spends a long time examining Tom and answering his questions. Nurse Anderson stays with him to help in the examination and to follow up points with Tom should this prove necessary. The surgical nurse manager also comes to see him. She is pleasant and a good listener and Tom finds it easy to talk to her.

On the Monday afternoon, Nurse Anderson records the following:

Observations

---

1 Physical state satisfactory – no abnormal blood pressure, pulse, respiration readings. Slight pyrexia: 37.6 °C. Wound not leaking.
2 30 ml water hourly by mouth as bowel sounds have been heard. Naso-gastric tube *in situ* in free drainage, aspirating four-hourly.
3 Intravenous infusion continued four-hourly – normal saline and dextrose.
4 Pethidine 50 mg, six-hourly if required.
5 Flatus passed, but bowels not opened. Urine passed and recorded.
6 Mobilised this morning, went for a short walk with physiotherapist.
7 Bathed – no skin abnormalities.
8 Nostril treated for soreness and naso-gastric tube readjusted to be more comfortable.

9 Intravenous infusion bandage readjusted for comfort.
10 Tom seems in control of his situation, asking specific questions.

What has happened so far to tell us how far Tom has got with his relationships with staff?

We can see that he is into a phase of exploitation because he has:

- passed the stage where he did not know what was happening to him;
- sought clarification about his situation;
- begun to identify with members of staff, particularly Staff Nurse Phillips, who admitted him and on whom he was dependent for support as well as a source of information;
- begun to share his problems with members of the health-care team;
- become involved in part of his own care – he is co-operating with members of staff;
- started to work through some of the issues surrounding his admission.

The relationships with particular members of staff are important to Tom: they are his bridge of reliability between one day and the next.

Phase of exploitation (2)

By Monday evening, Tom has been visited by two people, his brother and the minister. He was particularly pleased to see his brother, whom he likes and trusts. Tom's brother was given full information about his condition: this meant that the two brothers could share thoughts and feelings easily.

On Tuesday morning, about 7 a.m., Staff Nurse Phillips checks on Tom's condition and reports that things are going well. He has had a small bowel action and passed flatus. They talk about how long he will be in hospital and discuss how he has been coping with himself and members of staff. During the morning, he is seen by the consultant and registrar and the wound is inspected. The wound is cleaned, and sprayed with a dressing spray.

At lunchtime Nurse Anderson records the following:

Observations

1 Tom's naso-gastric tube has been removed; he is drinking normally.
2 Intravenous infusion discontinued.
3 Intravenous antibiotics discontinued.
4 Wound clean, sprayed but not re-dressed.
5 Bowels open once since this morning.
6 Urine passed, no bladder problems.
7 Fully mobile, being encouraged to walk as much as possible around the ward and to do deep-breathing exercises.
8 Washed in bathroom, will have a full bath this evening (at Tom's request).
9 Four-hourly temperature, pulse and respiration. Slight pyrexia: 37.6 °C.
10 Relating well to most people, at an adult-to-adult level, sometimes asks a number of questions covering similar ground on a regular basis. Says he is feeling better and less sore now that his tubes are out. Wants to know how long he will need to be off work.

Nurse Anderson feels that the plan of care is working well and Tom is taking more responsibility for himself.

Phase of resolution

By Tuesday evening, Tom is feeling tired and is in some discomfort. He feels that this is due to the fact that he was encouraged to walk around and that he has done too much. What pleases him is the small meal he has in the evening, some soup followed by a small amount of mashed potato, mince and gravy. He says that it tastes wonderful, and sees this as a sign that he is definitely getting better.

Staff Nurse Phillips sees Tom, discusses his progress and tries to check how anxious he is about his condition. He says that his anxiety lessens the more control he has; having the tubes out means he is free to walk around without being noticed so much.

Tom is visited by his brother who says that he is willing to stay a few days until Tom is 'on his feet again'. Staff Nurse Phillips feels that Tom has decreased his dependency on her. She sees that his brother is taking on the surrogacy role that has been her responsibility. She also realises that this freeing process involves both Tom and herself and that it needs talking through with him. She recognises that to free herself from the surrogacy role is more difficult than to initiate it. Any anxiety he might have about leaving hospital could be controlled by him being able to ask specific questions of people with whom he has good interpersonal relationships.

Tom sleeps well on Tuesday night, never really waking up. By Wednesday morning he is able with some assistance to get into the bath, and he has a cup of tea and some porridge for breakfast. By lunchtime, he has been seen by the registrar who has taken another blood sample to check his haemoglobin level and urea and electrolytes. He has his bowels open again and has passed a near-normal semi-formed stool. At lunch he has a small meal of soup, mashed potato and mince, followed by custard. Psychologically Tom seems to have gathered strength. He walks around without asking if he may; he has a wash when he wants it; he asks if he can visit the hospital chapel, which is arranged with the hospital chaplain.

During the afternoon of Wednesday, the registrar discusses with Tom the implications of going home. He thinks he could cope, but appears uncertain. When it is mentioned that a community nurse would come in every day for at least a week he seems happier at the suggestion. Tom discusses going home the following morning and arrangements are made with the community nurse to see him later on that day, Thursday. Tom's brother will collect him on Thursday morning at 9 a.m. He sleeps well on Wednesday night. On Thursday morning after breakfast his wound is re-checked, as is his temperature (37.6 °C).

His brother arrives with some outside clothes and while Tom is getting dressed, he finds out from the nurse in charge about an out-patient appointment and about the community nurse who will be coming to see Tom. Tom has been advised to stay off work for four weeks and to be seen by the surgeons before going back to work.

The feelings that Tom has about leaving hospital are generally positive. He is glad to be going home, to sleep in his own bed, but he will miss spending time with Staff Nurse Phillips, as she has provided an important support for him.

EVALUATION OF CARE

With Tom Richards, it is again useful to ask how well he coped with being in hospital. He needed to relate to someone very quickly, someone who was skilled in the care she could give and in listening.

His initial level of dependency and his methods of questioning are useful indications of how anxious he was about his condition and how he coped with it. Another point would be the ability of Tom to relate to other members of staff once he had established a reasonable relationship with the first significant person he had met. In this case he first made contact with Staff Nurse Phillips, but found talking with Staff Nurse Jones and Nurse Anderson less easy.

It could be true that Tom's coping behaviour was enhanced by his ability to relate well to Staff Nurse Phillips, which in turn substituted for the lack of psychological preparation for surgery. The shock and disbelief at his situation was to some extent reduced by a kind, effective relationship. This then provided Tom with an external focus for an internal conflict (Staff Nurse Phillips represented an external focus of comfort; shock and disbelief represented the internal conflict). The seesaw effects of internal conflict and external focus depended on Tom's ability to handle himself without being psychologically prepared, and on the relationship he made with a carer. The more established the relationship, the more influence Tom could have over his feelings, which in turn allowed him to be less influenced by his irrational thinking.

The care could also be evaluated by looking at Tom's capacity to cope with the thought of being able to go home. The observations of his verbal and non-verbal responses would be good indicators of how he felt about this. His actual response could then be viewed in comparison with what might have been a very different reaction. The important features in evaluation of Tom's care would be his response to being allowed to make an informed decision about himself, and his ability to go home from hospital.

For Staff Nurse Phillips the taking on of a surrogacy role had short- and long-term implications. Letting go of Tom's dependency on her, allowing him to become free and grow into adult behaviour patterns, was more difficult. She knew that by taking on this role she would have to cope with letting Tom move forward when he was recovering from surgery and that he too would have to allow this to happen (page 13).

QUESTIONS FOR DISCUSSION

1 In your opinion, how useful is Peplau's model in a surgical environment? What are the advantages and disadvantages?
   It would be helpful to work on your own at first and make notes. Follow this by meeting in a small group to discuss your ideas.

2 How well does Peplau's model enable general nurses to view the psychological care of patients within a physical nursing setting such as a surgical ward?

Use this question as a basis for a group discussion on the building of relationships and control of anxiety in patients with a physical illness.

EXERCISES

1 Following a period of supervised practice on a surgical ward, when you are together with a group of colleagues, try the following exercise.

Identify a patient with whom you have had some contact, a patient who was admitted as an emergency.

Write down your thoughts on how the patient coped with being admitted to hospital. Compare your notes with those of others in the group. Identify common aspects of such admissions, and comment on the responses in this case: 'did not cope well', 'coped very well', 'coped by crying' or 'coped by being angry'.

Discuss whether anxiety was associated with all the aspects you identified, and which aspect was associated with very high levels of anxiety. Then consider how in practice you could reduce the effect of high anxiety in a patient admitted as an emergency, and discuss what resources are at your disposal to enable you to do this.

You should allow about two hours for this exercise.

2 Consider how influential are the roles of stranger, surrogate, leader, teacher and counsellor in relation to a patient admitted into a surgical ward as an emergency. Think of a person you have nursed and try to identify which roles you adopted. List how easy or difficult these roles were for you to undertake.

Discuss your findings with a colleague and see how they compare with your partner's.

You should allow about one hour for this exercise.

CHAPTER EIGHT

Care studies: two people with mental health problems

The use of Peplau's model is useful in any branch of nursing, but in the field of mental health it is particularly so, because of its naturalness in using interpersonal skills as part of its essential framework. In this chapter, we meet two clients who each have a mental health problem, one relatively acute and the other longer-term.

MISS SYLVIA SHARP

Sylvia Sharp is 36 years old and works as an assistant in a public library. She enjoys her job, in general, and it seems to suit her personality to work in an atmosphere of quiet and control. Sylvia is a good-looking woman, but she has never been able to make a lasting social relationship. She therefore lived with her mother, who until recently had been well, but then fell down, broke her hip, and died in hospital, never really recovering from the fall.

The death of her mother devastated Sylvia, and she had to go to the general practitioner for help. The GP was very kind to Sylvia; he listened to her problems and anxieties and she felt supported by him. He gave her a mild tranquilliser so that she could feel calm enough to work during the day and to sleep at night, but he didn't feel that she needed an anti-depressant, as he thought that clinically she was more anxious than depressed. Following her mother's funeral, Sylvia gradually settled into some sort of routine. As she reflected on her mother's death, however, she realised that she was now alone in the world.

Sylvia began to lose the motivation to do anything, and going to work becamse a real struggle; she started to lose weight, as she stopped eating, and would cry a lot, often without apparent reason.

What frightened her, however, was the intense feeling of wanting to kill herself, and it was this that made her want to see the GP again. The doctor could see that Sylvia was in a poor physical and psychological state, so he asked a consultant from the local mental health unit to see her urgently. The consultant, Dr Brown, suggested that Sylvia be admitted to the unit for observation and care.

Within this particular unit the ward staff employ a 'key worker' system whereby a nurse is allocated to certain clients so that there can be some consistency of assessment and care. The key worker for Sylvia was Christine Knowles, a recently qualified psychiatric nurse. Christine now takes up the story.

'I was involved with Sylvia from the day of her admission. During the routine admission procedure, I could see that Sylvia was looking very sad and withdrawn. She found talking with me difficult and would take time in answering any questions I put to her. Sylvia had no real interest in the ward surroundings and did not appear to take in any information I gave her.

'Dr Brown examined Sylvia and had a long talk with her. Both of us discussed our observations about Sylvia at the ward staff meeting. It was decided to take Sylvia off her tranquillisers and to start her on Trimipramine to lift her depression. It was also agreed that I start to identify what short-term and longer-term goals would be useful to help Sylvia.'

PHASES OF THE NURSE–PATIENT RELATIONSHIP

Phase of orientation

Establishing a working relationship

On meeting for the first time, Christine and Sylvia are strangers, each one having her own separate ideas of what may happen, or not happen, during Sylvia's stay in hospital. The loss of her motivation for life and her depression are important factors for Christine to take into account at this stage of their relationship. These factors will directly affect Sylvia's expectations of improving.

Christine makes the following observations, documenting them in the nurse's notes:

Subjective observations	Objective observations
1 Sylvia appears to be very sad; she has a poor level of concentration; she has a sense of being uncertain; she seems to be unaware of her surroundings.	1 Sylvia is thin and has little appetite.
	2 She aches all over and complains that she sometimes feels sick.
2 She may be suicidal, but has not said anything about this.	3 She has had no period for two months.
3 She looks helpless, however, and she may feel as though her life is worthless.	4 She says that she is constipated.
	5 Facial expression: looks sad.
	6 She is not talking with anyone in the ward, unless she is approached.
	7 She cries without warning.

Christine discusses her observations with the ward manager and other staff, and it is agreed that a plan of care be drawn up, initially to establish contact with Sylvia so that a meaningful relationship can be started. The following goals are identified:

1 To pair Sylvia with other patients and get her to develop a friendship with them.
2 To identify whether the risk of Sylvia harming herself is very high.
3 To organise a programme of activity to help Sylvia reduce her isolation.
4 To keep the stress in Sylvia at a low level.
5 To provide adequate physical support to prevent Sylvia deteriorating.

Christine realises that the care she will provide must not be rushed: this would only agitate Sylvia and cause problems with their relationship.

A regime of care is established in which eating and drinking are encouraged, and hygiene measures can be carried out without haste. Sylvia is given time to talk and relate to Christine.

Phase of identification

Providing a deeper relationship

Forty-eight hours after admission Sylvia seems to have settled into the unit. She remains withdrawn and needs active help and encouragement to wash, dress, eat and drink. Sylvia goes to the toilet and has her bowels open. Her levels of awareness and her ability to concentrate remain low. During the next two days, Christine has been off duty, so the relationship established with her and Sylvia is still at an embryonic stage. Christine feels, however, that some progress will be made over the next few days as she will not be going off duty for another six days.

Over the next forty-eight hours, Christine works with Sylvia. With difficulty Christine gets Sylvia to talk more about herself and what led up to her needing admission. She finds out that Sylvia has no relatives alive, and that the loss of her mother was more than she could bear. (Christine notes that Sylvia not only cries when talking about her mother, but also seems to 'come alive', putting her hands into fists and moving her arms about; she notes too that her facial expression changes.)

Sylvia says, 'I wouldn't be missed if I wasn't here in the world.' This comment is taken seriously by the nursing staff as a possible cue to ideas of suicide.

In her notes, Christine documents the following:

Notes

Sylvia has started to talk with me about her present coping mechanisms, and is talking a little more about how she is feeling. I feel that my relationship with her is now becoming more trusting and meaningful and that she is beginning to identify with me. She talks about no one missing her if she wasn't around; I feel this is a reference to her feeling suicidal, and the fact that she has told me this makes me feel she is trusting me more – and testing me out, perhaps – and that she wants help.

Christine also notes the following:

Subjective observations	Objective observations
1 Sylvia seems to be identifying with me, most of the time.	1 She is eating and drinking fairly well.
2 She seems to indicate that she is a worthless person.	2 She is taking her medication without difficulty.
3 She is possibly very angry that her mother has died, because she has been abandoned.	3 She sleeps badly at times; she usually wakes up early in the morning.
4 She probably relies heavily on people to provide her with any self-esteem.	4 She is starting to listen to music on the radio.
	5 She is not talking very much with other clients in the unit.

In regard to the subjective observation that Sylvia is identifying with Christine most of the time, the staff nurse would have to consider what roles Sylvia is putting Christine into. The role of leader, where decisions are being made for Sylvia, seems very likely; so does the role of surrogate, because she rarely made decisions without her mother's permission.

How should Christine respond? In order to capitalise on their developing closeness, Christine needs to address with Sylvia how her mother influenced her, both in social contacts and with people where there was the potential for a deeper relationship. She could then refer to the relationship between Sylvia and herself, and note how dependent Sylvia is on her. Knowing that the nurse–patient relationship is professionally led, with a definite cut-off point, Christine has to consider how Sylvia can maintain a good level of self-esteem outside hospital (pages 36–9). The role of friend that Christine is developing may have to be continued in the community for some time until Sylvia adapts to living and working normally again.

Christine talks about Sylvia with Dr Brown and the other members of the health care team. He interviews Sylvia and relates his impressions to the unit staff. He feels that Sylvia may be angry with her mother for dying; her mother was a powerful person in Sylvia's life and this anger may stem from a feeling of being abandoned.

It is decided to continue the original programme of short-term goals with Sylvia, but because the phase of identification has now been established, some longer-term goals could be discussed with Sylvia as well. The following plan is therefore identified:

> 1 To continue to develop a deeper relationship.
> 2 To watch for signs of Sylvia harming herself.
> 3 To keep her involved in ward activities.
> 4 To continue to support her in maintaining a reasonable state of health.
> 5 To observe her sleep patterns.
> 6 To aim to improve her self-esteem by working through issues of importance in her life.

Over the next few days, Christine works with Sylvia, and the relationship between them deepens. Sylvia shares some of her personal history and relates that she has always had a problem relating to others and that she blames herself a lot when something goes wrong. She also relates that she rarely made decisions for herself, without her mother's permission.

Phase of exploitation

Learning how to cope

Over the next seven days, Sylvia begins to show signs of improvement. She is eating quite well and is putting on weight. She continues to sleep badly at times, but generally feels that she is developing a better sleep pattern. She washes and dresses herself spontaneously and goes to the toilet regularly to have her bowels open. Sylvia keeps quite active during the day, but sometimes seems to be reluctant to join in some ward activities.

The ward staff meet regularly and discuss her progress. Christine makes the following notes about Sylvia:

Subjective observations	Objective observations
1 Sylvia seems to be relating to me well.	1 She is eating well and putting on weight.
2 She seems still to be angry about feeling helpless in her life.	2 Her sleep pattern is better, but she still has early-wakening problems now and again.
3 I feel she wants to be more comfortable when making decisions for herself.	3 She is taking medication easily.

80

Subjective observations	Objective observations
4 She could become agitated if we expect her to make her own decisions too quickly and without proper support. 5 She is probably rather dependent on me.	4 She washes and dresses herself. 5 She is relating to one or two selected clients and staff only. 6 Facial expression: she looks less sad than when she was admitted.

It is agreed that the plan of care developed in the phase of identification should be further developed, by getting Sylvia gradually to take on decisions in her life in a supportive framework. Sylvia is encouraged to take some exercise – walking outside with a member of staff – and to visit some local shops. As no one has visited her, it is gently suggested that someone from work could come to see her. Christine notes the following: 'When it was suggested that Sylvia had a visit from colleagues in the library, she became rather anxious and expressed some doubt as to whether they would want to come.' This seems to Christine to indicate that Sylvia is still having a problem with her self-esteem and that thoughts of suicide are possibly very real. It takes some time for Sylvia to agree to a visit, and the first meeting with her immediate boss seems strained, but subsequent visits get easier.

It is also noticed that Sylvia is concentrating more easily when talking with staff and clients and that she is less withdrawn in herself. She is invited to take part in an assertion group which is being run in the unit, the aim being to help her cope with decision-making and to start a link that can be continued as an out-patient once she has been discharged.

A major step forward is when Sylvia has a period. This is the first one she has experienced in three months, and she relates that she feels more like an adult again.

Christine discusses the relationship that Sylvia has with her. She realises that the process of 'letting go' of the bond they have will probably be a difficult one, although Christine has never felt that she has over-identified with Sylvia.

Phase of resolution

Being in control

After being in the unit for just over four weeks, Sylvia has improved both mentally and physically. Her mood has elevated and the anti-depressant medication is apparently working. She remains shy but is able to ask for things. She indicates that she feels more is happening in her life now and that things are not so black. Physically she is stronger and her sleep pattern has improved.

An arrangement is made where she goes home for a day, with Christine. She copes quite well with this: this suggests that she would like to be dependent on Christine as a surrogate mother. Dr Brown discusses with Sylvia the possibility of going home for a weekend and being visited by the staff. Sylvia copes with this well and two weeks later is discharged. Visits from the community psychiatric nurse are arranged and Sylvia continues as an out-patient to have regular sessions in the assertion group. A follow-up appointment is made to see Dr Brown. The anti-depressant therapy is gradually reduced and Sylvia starts work again in the library some three months after her admission.

EVALUATION OF CARE

The relationship with Sylvia when she was acutely depressed could, without any exaggeration, be considered a lifeline. The problem of Sylvia harming herself remains real, as does the fear of the unknown.

In evaluating the care given, the indications of progress could be seen in the nursing notes and other documentation. Documenting changes in mood and behaviour provides a good measure of Sylvia's progress and is therefore crucial as a monitor. The actual outcomes of care could be compared with the aims in the plan of care (page 80): did care succeed in helping Sylvia's forward movement of personality from the phase of exploitation to the phase of resolution? Another consideration is the alteration of Christine's role as a leader and surrogate: from the more directive leadership style, Christine could move to a more democratic style (see pages 25–6). The freeing process for Sylvia – her willingness to undertake this responsibility – would be another cue to her development into the phase of resolution. Other points for consideration would be Sylvia's progress in initiating communication with others around her and how well these contacts went.

82

Many issues remain for Sylvia, not least the feeling that she needs to find at least one real person outside hospital with whom she can have an enduring social relationship. She may also require longer-term help to see why she feels about herself as she does, and what happened in her childhood years to make her behave as she does. However, the framework of nursing and medical care she received as an in-patient has given her the opportunity to begin looking at these longer-term problems.

MRS AGNES HUNT

Agnes Hunt is married and aged 41. She has three children by a previous marriage; she divorced her first husband when she was 36. She remarried two years later. When she was a child, Agnes was physically abused by her father and like her two brothers she felt that she was never loved or wanted by her parents. Leaving home was easy for her to do, but making a life for herself in the world was difficult. She felt very resentful of her parents because of this, and felt that they forced her to leave home. Her three children – John aged 22, Clara aged 20, and Simon aged 18 – are all living away from home, so Agnes is now living with her husband, Fred, only.

During her first marriage, Agnes had problems bringing up the children. Her first husband, Alan, would often hit her and the children and so the relationship was never on a sound footing. Agnes suffered from periods of depression which were treated with anti-depressants. Usually this treatment worked but sometimes Agnes would need admission to hospital because she felt suicidal.

When her depression was under control, she would become quite aggressive and behave irresponsibly. It was a combination of all these factors that led to the ending of her first marriage. When Agnes remarried, things seemed to go well with her new husband, but as time went on she felt that Fred was trying to harm her: to protect herself she would frequently attack him. She attended a mental health clinic regularly, and it was decided that she should have contact with the community mental health team. A community psychiatric nurse called Steve Petersfield has now been asked to work with Agnes and to monitor her behaviour.

Steve arranges to meet with Agnes in her home. Fred is also at home. Fred stays out of the front room where Steve and Agnes are talking, making an excuse to be doing something else around the house. Steve introduces himself and after some initial talking about her history asks Agnes what her present difficulties are.

'I don't know what I should tell you,' says Agnes. 'I have had the same problems for years, so why you should be involved with me now I just don't know.' Steve recognises that Agnes is anxious when she is saying this and feels that she may be showing covert hostility towards him. Agnes continues, 'I am feeling well at the moment and I am irritated easily by people asking me questions.' Again, Steve feels some resentment and hostility towards him. He comments that he recognises that she doesn't know him and that he appreciates her feelings, but asks her to say, if she will, a little more about what is happening to her at the moment. 'I love Fred, he understands me, but I feel so bad when I get cross with him and hit him. I think he wants to hurt me sometimes, like poison me – I am convinced he wants to get rid of me because I treat him like my father did or my first husband, Alan.' This raises the possibility that Agnes has set up a replication of these poorly understood earlier relationships with men, because she talks about how she treats Fred.

Steve spends some time with Agnes and notices that she is showing unpredictable and aggressive behaviour towards Fred and others who get to know her well.

PHASES OF THE NURSE–PATIENT RELATIONSHIP

Phase of orientation

Steve makes the following notes about Agnes in addition to the family and personal history:

Subjective observations	Objective observations
1 Agnes get angry with people because she has never had the opportunity to trust and be wanted on a consistent basis.	1 Agnes shows signs of being very anxious when talking about herself or her family.
2 She loses her temper, perhaps when she feels that she is not controlling a situation.	2 She has suspicions about her husband wanting to hurt her.
3 Agnes may have a lot of hostility towards men she has known and may not be able	3 She has suppressed anger towards her husband.
	4 Fred seems to be controlled by Agnes.
	5 There is a risk of Agnes being misunderstood by people.

Subjective observations	Objective observations
to trust them even if they are kind. 4 She expects to be treated badly by men and experiences anxiety when this expectation is not met, for example if they are kind instead of hurtful to her.	

Steve discusses his visit with the community mental health team. From the debate certain points arise:

- Agnes will take time to accept Steve's role as a stranger and she may misunderstand what is said to her. Steve will need to discuss with Agnes the level of dependency each may have on the other and how important this aspect of their relationship will be.
- She remains suspicious of people and believes that Fred wants to harm her. This makes her behave aggressively towards him.
- She has been physically and psychologically hurt by people close to her in the past, making it hard for her to develop meaningful relationships.
- Steve's initial relationship with Agnes has not been well established. Fred has not been seen, and his thoughts and feelings about Agnes have not been explored. Therefore, it is important to try to see Agnes and Fred together.
- Agnes has a history of mental health problems.

A plan of care is organised. During the phase of orientation the goals will be short-term:

1 To help Agnes recognise angry feelings and to encourage her to express them in a constructive way.
2 To be available as much as possible in this early phase and to respond quickly to Agnes should she ask for help.
3 To recognise that the nurse–client relationship will take time to develop.

Phase of identification

Steve sees Agnes twice more over a period of four days and has some opportunity to see Fred. Steve feels that Fred is frightened of what Agnes could do to him, although he will not talk about it too much. The discussions with Agnes centre around her feelings about trusting people and it becomes clear that Agnes does not want to trust because she is frightened of becoming hurt or rejected. When this happens, she becomes angry and defensive and closes off from people. Steve notes that Agnes is probably very vulnerable as an individual and has had some bad experiences in the past. As she finds it difficult to talk through her feelings, she becomes hostile.

Steve also notes the following:

Subjective observations	Objective observations
1 Agnes finds it difficult to communicate her feelings.	1 Agnes is talking with me more easily. She is not showing any overt hostility.
2 She worries about what people think of her.	2 She seems orientated to time and place, and does not have any problems remembering events.
3 She wants to express warmth and kindness but finds this difficult because it is something she has rarely experienced.	3 She gets upset if she talks about her lack of trust in others.
4 She wants lasting relationships, but uses aggression to manipulate people into keeping in contact with her.	4 There is no evidence of her wanting to injure herself.

The community team recognise that Steve must maintain a consistent calm approach and remain available. Agnes is beginning to confront herself a little more by talking in more depth about trusting others.

Over the next three months, Steve visits Agnes regularly and on some occasions, when he is not at work, talks to Fred. Most times Agnes talks about trusting people and her feelings towards Fred, her children, and her mother and father. She relates that both her parents are alive, but other than a postcard at Christmas she never hears from them. The children do not hear from their grandparents, either.

After two and a half months of talking with Agnes, Steve feels that he has established a reasonably good relationship and that Agnes is making an effort to communicate more effectively and attempting to keep her aggression under control. At times she is unable to discuss things rationally and gets anxious, but most times she succeeds in getting her thoughts and feelings across. From the point of view of nursing care, Steve feels that the phase of identification has been reasonably established.

Phase of exploitation

Over the next two months Steve maintains a regular contact with his client. He discusses his progress regularly with other community staff and in particular the following observations:

Subjective observations	Objective observations
1 Agnes seems to be less hostile and interacts at a more meaningful level with people around her.	1 She is talking more easily and finds questions less intimidating.
2 Her level of dependency on me is high.	2 She looks forward to seeing me on a regular basis.
3 She will have problems taking on more responsibility for her behaviour without support.	3 There have been no recent episodes of Agnes hitting Fred.
4 She is probably very worried about relapsing again, as she feels she is generally doing well.	4 She seems to accept that she is socially vulnerable. She wants to be able to get over this present problem.

Steve plans to develop Agnes's individuality and levels of responsibility, but realises the road to achieving this will be long and hard.

The level of dependency that Agnes has on Steve becomes evident to him when in one conversation she asks, 'You are still going to be around here next year?' and 'Have you any plans for moving away?' Once Steve has answered that he has no immediate plans, she talks in some depth about her relationship with her previous husband, relating how cruel and uncaring he was. When asked why she wanted to know about Steve moving away, she replies that there is no particular reason.

87

Steve feels that Agnes is checking how far she could trust him and he realises that the dependency she has is still an important issue to be addressed.

Phase of resolution

The difficulty for Agnes is that she has had a long-term problem in coping with trusting relationships and it is hard to change her expectations of others, especially now. Her history indicates that she is a socially vulnerable person who is having to learn to change her lifestyle. During her childhood she was not loved as an individual and she was powerless coping with her father, who beat her frequently. This situation continued in her first marriage and in some ways Agnes did not expect warmth. She was suspicious of warmth when it did occur, and could only imagine that warmth had a 'price'.

Very gradually, over the next three months, Steve discussed with Agnes and Fred the need to love and respect each other, and the fact that Agnes could relieve her aggression by constructive discussions. Like Steve, the community team felt that periodic support would be necessary for Agnes. The years of pain and lack of trust could not be resolved in a space of nine months. Steve notes the following points, however:

Subjective/objective observations

---

1 Agnes's feelings of hostility towards her father remain much the same. She will need to explore this area carefully as it will affect how she improves in the future.
2 Agnes seems to agree that she is now better able to cope with her feelings generally.
3 She seems more in control now than nine months ago.
4 She recognises the need to express – to put into words rather than act out – how she feels when she gets hostile, angry or frustrated, although she knows that she may fail to do this well.
5 She remains worried that she may regress and start to demonstrate aggression again, and she is not certain how she would cope with that if it happened.
6 Her feeling that Fred is trying to harm her has gone.

Agnes is offered follow-up help if she needs it. She has now had one reasonable relationship (significantly, with a man), where some of

88

her strong feelings have been discussed. In this sense she has moved towards being a more complete human being.

EVALUATION OF CARE

For Steve the role of stranger in the early phases of care was important. Agnes was reluctant to talk with him at first and her growth cue was to accept his friendship. What is important is the identification and resolution of problems generated by Agnes. The depth of the initial relationship is essential if these problems are to be satisfactorily explored. In the early phase of their relationship the active–passive alliance was evident (see page 37); this was followed by the co-operative alliance in the later phases of care (see page 38). This change in co-operation could be seen as Agnes was going through to the phases of identification and exploitation.

The other main problem for Steve is what role Agnes will now try to place him in. Her experiences with men have not been happy ones, and she is used to manipulating situations to reduce her feelings of vulnerability. Steve could be taking on a surrogate role, where he provides enough stability for Agnes to say how anxious she feels. The success of this initial activity can be judged from Agnes's willingness to allow Steve to act in the roles of counsellor and teacher. This growth cue would be a sign of her beginning to use the relationship in an adult-to-adult way, and accepting the process of resolution in which she begins to free herself from excessive dependency.

Within a community setting, nurses work independently, although they have the back-up of a mental health team. Yet it is on the basis of the face-to-face interactions that decisions on how people are progressing must be made. With clients who have a mental health problem, it is helpful to evaluate care under various headings:

Mental state Here the nurse could look for changes in someone who is hallucinated, deluded, or confused. In addition she could look for disturbances of mood and memory lapses.

Behaviour The areas of evaluation could be the reduction of phobias, compulsive and ritualistic behaviour, drink or drug problems, self-harm, and aggression.

Interpersonal problems The nurse could evaluate the effect of a relationship with partners, other family members and professionals.

Psychological and social problems Areas for evaluating progress could be the reduction of anxiety and social isolation.

Physical problems This might include menstrual problems, sleep patterns, appetite, weight, and physical tension in the body.

Many points for evaluation of care in mental health problems are not measurable. The careful documentation of observations is therefore very important, as are the points raised in discussions with other professionals. Peplau's model offers a framework in which to monitor change taking place and provides a basis for accurate assessment, planning, implementation and evaluation of care.

QUESTIONS FOR DISCUSSION

1 What roles do others (such as senior nurses and doctors) play in the supervision of your practice, in helping you evaluate the effectiveness of nursing care?
   This question can be used by individuals or as a group exercise.
2 What are the benefits of using Peplau's model of nursing with clients who have a mental health problem?
   Use this as a group question.
3 What are the short- and long-term consequences of taking on a surrogate role with someone who is vulnerable and potentially dependent?
   Work on this question and talk to others about your ideas.
4 Is the freeing process in the phase of resolution as difficult for the nurse as it is for the patient? Is the process more difficult for people who have mental health problems rather than physical problems?
   This would be a very useful question to ask following clinical practice in a mental health or handicap unit, or in community care, especially as a group exercise.

PART III

Critique of the model

CHAPTER NINE

The axiology of Peplau's model

The word 'axiology' stems from the Greek *axios*, which means 'worthy'. Axiology is the study of values and value judgements. This chapter looks at the values inherent in Peplau's model of nursing.

USING PEPLAU'S MODEL

A model of nursing is a general collection of ideas or concepts that form a framework which may help nurses to make decisions on how how to care for someone. A nursing model is therefore produced to assist us in what we do: the model is useful only if we can subscribe to its ideas and the values implicit in the various paradigms.

Peplau's model is an early attempt to show how nurses might look at care provision. Peplau was one of the first people to ask how nurses do what they do. She developed her concepts from a psychoanalytical paradigm: she focused on the development of a therapeutic relationship as the important process, and sought to provide a relationship that would work towards the person remaining healthy. To do this effectively meant that nurses would have to learn to use the anxiety experienced by a patient or relative to help them understand what the problems were and how those problems could be dealt with. Using the relationship in this way, by educating, collaborating, and being a therapist, the nurse would be able to empathise with the patient's problems. Consequently, both the nurse and the patient would learn and grow. Peplau saw that patients would experience problems if these needs were not met, either because the anxiety was too high or because the tensions in the patient caused frustration and conflict.

Peplau's model is about caring for someone by interaction: it is therefore reasonable to describe it as a developmental model rather than a systems model. Peplau sees people as unique; her model reflects phases of care that are broad enough to be tailored to each individual. The patient is also seen as an equal partner in the care that is being explored and provided; the care should be an opportunity for the patient to learn about himself. To care for the patient well, the nurse should be mature enough to cope with the dynamics of the interpersonal process, and be prepared to learn about herself as she interacts.

To be relevant in practice, Peplau's model has to be used within the social contexts of both the nurse and the patient; it must be considered in terms of how supportive it is in helping a patient view his present state of health. If we look at the characteristics of an interactionist model, as discussed by Benoliel (1977) and Heiss (1976), we can see that social acts, relationship-building, role and self-concept all impinge on some of the features of Peplau's model. However, the hallmarks of a developmental model of nursing as discussed by Chin (1980) are very relevant to Peplau's thinking. These characteristics include growth, and being able to progress and develop a potential for living a fuller life. In terms of putting Peplau's model into practice the nurse should be aware of these characteristics: unless the nurse can accept them, value them and use them, the practice of care within the framework of Peplau's model is difficult and perhaps impossible. For example, when a nurse and patient meet they are strangers. The nurse takes on different roles as the relationship grows, which suit her and (it is hoped) help the patient; they get to know and adjust to each other. When the nurse takes on a surrogate role, this fulfils a need in the patient, who wants a substitute around to help him through some area of difficulty. The nurse must remember, however, that taking on these different roles has many effects on the patient, and on herself. As Peplau's model uses this focus as the main thrust of caring, the nurse must be able to manage the emotions that emanate from her taking up new roles, both in herself and the patient.

The value of Peplau's model in different settings

The examples of patient care in Part II of this book give an idea of how Peplau's model can be used in different settings. Two points arise.

1 The phases of interpersonal relationship – orientation, identification, exploitation and resolution – are relevant in getting to know a

patient. They therefore allow the nurse to be able to assess, plan, implement and evaluate care.

2 The *skills* involved in looking after someone – in paediatrics, in care of the elderly, in medical, surgical, mental health or mental handicap nursing, in hospital or community nursing – are not affected by the phases of the interpersonal relationship. The phases are relevant in determining how the technical skills should be introduced to the patient.

The management of anxiety in the patient

As Peplau's model is based on the premise of a psychoanalytical base, anxiety is a central theme in the care of the patient. I have cared for many patients over the years, many of whom were able to relate to me and I to them; practically all of them have experienced anxiety about themselves and their condition. It is part of the human experience of being unwell. It is therefore present in one form or another and shows itself in different ways. How it is perceived by the patient and by the nurse depends on their maturity and individual make-up. As each person is unique, it is difficult to predict how someone is going to react in any given situation, but the phases of care described by Peplau afford *some* control over this. For example, the anxiety levels of a newly admitted patient may be high because of the fear of the unknown: this anxiety can be reduced by getting to know the person and allowing him to talk through the problems he feels are ahead of him. Peplau is saying that a nurse can, by developing a relationship, get to know the patient and his feelings. She is saying also that the nurse should expect the unexpected.

The management of anxiety in a patient is a skilled process, because its expression is unpredictable. A useful step is to accept that anxiety exists in everyone who is ill and that if it is to be managed it needs to be explored. This raises an important point: is it desirable for a patient to experience some anxiety while he is being cared for? This may seem a strange question to ask, yet it is an important one to address when using Peplau's model. When someone is ill and needs help, they have many thoughts and feelings about themselves; they may be worried about the illness they have, or what it will mean to them in the future. They may be concerned about whether they are going to get better or not, and whether the treatment they need will be effective or painful. They may have concerns about whom they can trust, about who will give them answers to the questions they have. The anxiety caused by such

95

Figure 9.1 Anxiety and control

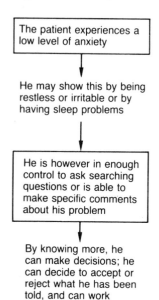

The patient experiences a low level of anxiety	*Anxiety should be expected in anyone who is ill*
He may show this by being restless or irritable or by having sleep problems	*Other signs of anxiety may be present, such as being defensive, being awkward, crying, thinking inwardly*
He is however in enough control to ask searching questions or is able to make specific comments about his problem	*The patient has enough awareness to realise that by asking questions or commenting he can understand his situation more easily*
By knowing more, he can make decisions; he can decide to accept or reject what he has been told, and can work through some of his thoughts and feelings in a constructive way	*The patient will rely on the nurse or others in the health team to give him time to do this: he will also need to feel that he is being accepted as a unique person who is worth being listened to*

thoughts and feelings determines how they behave. The deeper feelings the patient has will become known to a nurse only if the relationship is a sound one. As Peplau's model uses the approach of an interpersonal relationship, the anxiety and defensiveness of the patient is confronted. Anxiety levels will diminish if the patient talks about his problems to someone he trusts. By working through a problem the patient becomes aware of possible answers to help him resolve the conflict he is experiencing. A low level of anxiety may make the patient ask questions, but he is still in control because his anxiety is manageable. If the level of anxiety becomes high, the patient's self-awareness becomes less manageable; he worries excessively and cannot gain control. He is not able to ask appropriate questions to help him elucidate how he is going to cope in future. This can be shown diagrammatically (Figures 9.1 and 9.2).

When a patient is anxious, it is therapeutic to use the energy produced by that anxiety in a constructive way. The anxiety unlocks some of the deeper feelings that the patient wants to discuss: by

Figure 9.2 Anxiety and no control

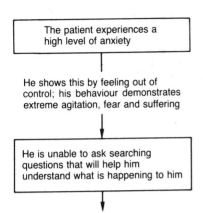

| The patient experiences a high level of anxiety | The patient feels that his situation is neither controllable nor bearable |

He shows this by feeling out of control; his behaviour demonstrates extreme agitation, fear and suffering

He uses defensive behaviour to cope, maybe rationalising or denying his situation: his anger comes out aggressively, which causes others to behave defensively; he has lost his ability to be self-aware and cannot formulate searching questions

He is unable to ask searching questions that will help him understand what is happening to him

His needs are not being met or resolved; he finds it difficult to co-operate and be able to listen

The staff cope on a very short-term basis: time spent with the patient is emotionally draining, and the patient is not an equal partner in the care process

accepting it, exploring it, and working through how he can come to terms with it, important progress can be made. Providing the nurse and patient have a good working relationship the level of anxiety experienced by the patient can be used to help cope with future events. The hurt to someone in doing this is small compared with the hurt experienced by someone who has not addressed the issues at all. The emotional hurt felt by a patient experiencing high anxiety is far more damaging than the process of exploring anxiety when it can be managed by him. In practice as the level of anxiety increases in someone, the questions become more searching until a point is reached where the anxiety takes over, and the questioning becomes less controlled and specific.

A framework for thinking

The value of Peplau's model is its use as a framework in which a working, trusting relationship can be built up with a patient. The model is flexible enough to allow its use in different clinical settings. The success of its use therefore depends on whether nurses can agree that the model is something that can be used in clinical practice, so it is imperative that the principles implicit in the model are understood – if they are not, the principles cannot be put into action. This is true of any model of nursing, for a concept developed in someone's mind and set out on paper must be scrutinised carefully as it is put into practice. A major deficiency in nursing today is the lack of understanding of what a nursing model is there to do. If a model is put into a clinical situation without its users properly knowing how it can be used, it is unlikely to benefit the practice of nursing care.

POTENTIAL DIFFICULTIES IN USING PEPLAU'S MODEL

No conceptual model of nursing is perfect. There are drawbacks to every framework devised, and only its use over a period of time can identify its strengths and weaknesses. This situation means that others can explore how models can be improved and developed. As the world changes, new thinking about care is inevitable; as nursing grows as a profession, the discussions we have about caring become part of that growth.

We have considered in this book the value of using a humanistic interactional model. So what are the potential difficulties in using Peplau's model in the world of nursing today?

The use of a humanistic model

Peplau's model uses the core concept that interpersonal relationships are vital. When words are exchanged, so are feelings. This model, then, will produce emotion in the carers. As the patient wants the framework to explore and understand himself, the nurse is carried along the same path of thinking. This is not always easy for the nurse, who has to cope with the feelings generated in her about herself as well as about the patient.

If a nurse is uncertain of her role in this relationship, the levels of anxiety she feels may become difficult to manage. The importance of the nurse, in the Peplau model, is in providing adequate therapeutic support, and it is crucial to this that she feels confident in her ability to communicate effectively. The model requires highly developed skills of communication, which need to be taught well and discussed in depth in the nurse's basic educational programme: if this has not been done, the use of Peplau's model in clinical practice is in doubt.

The use of time

An essential ingredient in using Peplau's model is the building up of a relationship such that the nurse and patient work together. It is expected that the patient will become involved in his care and will have some equality in the relationship. This requires time.

In some instances the model is ideal in providing a framework for thinking. For patients who have a mental health problem, where contact is usually intense and enduring, the time is there to develop this relationship as the patient needs care over a number of weeks. This is usually true also of situations in the community where there is always an extended one-to-one relationship between a community nurse and the patient.

Time is more of a problem in establishing a relationship in areas of nursing where patients are admitted and discharged in a short space of time, perhaps 24–48 hours. Mechanistic care can easily be provided; relationship-building is more of a problem. To some extent this will remain a difficulty until alternative ways of managing patients are developed, such as primary nursing, key-worker roles, and follow-up care. Until pilot schemes have been tried to see how this would work, time remains a problem in using such a humanistic model.

The use of counselling skills

When patients are thinking things through, working on possible answers to a problem, or needing guidance and support, the carer needs an adequate understanding of how counselling will assist this process.

Counselling relies on the effective use of communication skills. The nurse needs to be able to provide an understanding environment in which the patient can feel safe to explore areas of concern, anxiety or difficulty. He can then identify possible answers to a problem. Counselling is *not* about giving advice, but about providing an opportunity for a patient to sort things out in his mind and to draw some reasonable conclusions. The relatives of patients too may need guidance and support in order to co-operate in the care a patient receives.

Counselling is a difficult skill to acquire. It requires a person to be educated in the fundamentals of using listening, speaking, questioning and reflecting in particular ways. Yet the Peplau model relies on the use of counselling as one of the major skills that a nurse *must* have. Not everyone who gives nursing care feels comfortable counselling, where it is the patient who has control in the situation. The only control the nurse exercises is in directing the discussion by the questions she asks. Less experienced carers may shift control in their own favour by resorting to advising.

Providing a network of support for staff

The patient dependency studies in Part II of this book show the potential value in providing meaningful, fulfilling care, but this makes great emotional demands of the carer. The nurse will herself need to be supported. If support is not forthcoming there will be a greater need to feel secure in building relationships with patients. Time has to be invested in staff support: nurses need times when clinical practice can be discussed. The ideal may be the use of a nurse consultant who has the background skills required, but as yet this system of support is rare in many nursing disciplines. Although support is needed in any nursing situation, it is especially important when using humanistic skills within a model, where interpersonal relationships form the core of nursing practice. The need for staff support is now well recognised, but its implementation in the clinical situation is patchy. The Peplau model raises awareness of the need for a sound staff network of support: it is difficult to practise when isolated from the support and guidance of other staff.

The provision of adequate support means that the skills of supervision, teaching, and counselling have to be taught and discussed with all staff. Professional development for trained nurses to take on these reponsibilities therefore needs to be provided. Nursing staff may otherwise have difficulty in committing themselves to using Peplau's model: in any humanistic approach to care, the nurse is provided only with a framework to give direction – the model does not prescribe how the nurse should act, so a support network is essential.

DOCUMENTING NURSING PRACTICE

Over the years, a number of different ideas have been generated on how nursing care should be documented. Like models of nursing, none of these is perfect. Some provide better structures than others, but no one system will suit everybody. The progress that has been made from a medical model to nursing models has meant that people have started to think about the *process* of nursing care.

It takes several years using documents to see where their strengths and weaknesses lie. Hospitals in the same group often use different documents, which perhaps suggests that documentation, like Peplau's model, is dynamic and must be changed and adapted to benefit everyone.

It is difficult to fit a model's concepts into an existing documentation structure. In humanistic models it is hard to be mechanistic, and yet it is important to work with a documentation structure over a period of time: this helps keep costs down and assists staff by giving them some stability. In Part II, the patient dependency studies, structure was kept to a minimum: this was to allow the reader to think about the concepts of the model and to avoid a mechanistic presentation of the material. This highlights the potential difficulties in writing down what has been covered with a patient while using such a model as Peplau.

One approach is to see how the phases of interaction match the process of nursing (Figure 9.3). Another is to have lined paper on which the phase of care is noted, following by sub-headings of assessing, planning, implementing and evaluating care, as illustrated in Figure 9.4. A third possibility is to use plain paper on which the nurse writes her notes about the phase of interaction and care she has given. It is possible to employ a Kardex system specifically designed to be flexible in what requires documenting, or to design a package to be used within a computerised system of documenting nursing care. To record both subjective and objective observations about a patient requires considerable thought, however, and this is a potential problem when representing Peplau's model.

EVALUATION OF CARE

Like other models, Peplau's approach to managing nursing care requires public scrutiny. To evaluate how effective someone has been in looking after an ill person one needs suitable evaluation tools. The model itself is not measurable, because it discusses nursing in broad terms, so theories of nursing arising from using the model must be explored if the model itself is to be tested.

The evaluation of care is seldom done often enough or well enough; evaluation is an aspect of care that has not been investigated thoroughly: the research nurse is well placed to confront this

Figure 9.3 The phase of orientation within a document using the nursing process

Phase of care	Assessment of care	Planning care	Implementing care	Evaluating care
Orientation Mr Jones is anxious about his admission. A relationship must be built up.	Restless and asking questions.	Needs time to have his situation explained to him. Aim to reduce his anxiety levels.	Time given 30 minutes: spent with Mr Jones answering questions and listening to his worries.	Appears less restless. Seems to have his anxiety lessened. Review tomorrow.
Mr Jones is concerned about his operation tomorrow.	Needs to have an opportunity to sit and talk this through.	Check his concerns about the operation. Provide information if wanted.	Mr Jones talked about his concerns. Identified that pain following his operation is causing his most concern. Discussed with him the need to talk to the doctor as well as to me. I need to see the doctor as well about Mr Jones's concern.	Spoke to the doctor. Will talk carefully with the patient about post-operative pain. Need to follow up Mr Jones later today to see whether his concern has been reduced.

Figure 9.4 Care plan

Patient's name: _____ Hospital no.: _____

Date: _____ Phase of the relationship: _____

Assessment of patient's needs

_____

_____

_____

_____

Plan of care

_____

_____

_____

_____

Implementation of care

_____

_____

_____

_____

Evaluation of care

_____

_____

_____

_____

deficiency. In the case of an interactional model, *feelings* about care have to be considered. Feelings are, in fact, a major tool by which nurses assess patients' needs. Yet they can be measured most proficiently only by methods of self-assessment and self-awareness.

A way forward, to reduce this problem, might be to use a psychological scale of patient dependency that works alongside, and is integrated with, a scale of physical dependency. In Peplau's model, it might be helpful to use a scale of dependency linked to the level of anxiety the patient is experiencing, which in turn dictates the amount of time needed with that patient. The use of measurement in nursing a patient using an interactional approach, where parameters of care are changing, is a difficulty which has yet to be overcome.

SUMMARY

The model of care produced by Peplau provides us with an opportunity to develop nursing as an interactional process, so allowing both the nurse and the patient to identify care. Although nursing in practice is seen as helping someone improve their quality of life, Peplau saw the importance of developing a focus on health-related issues. The model represents the use of anxiety as a means whereby the carer can assist the patient in identifying his problems and how these might be handled. In this way the patient's tension and concerns can be kept at manageable levels.

As Peplau's model puts such importance upon the relationship, the carer also has to be aware of her own feelings and values. The involvement of the nurse in this relationship implies a need for her to be adequately supported. In this model it is appreciated that each patient is unique, and the nurse should therefore see the dignity and worth experienced by the patient as individual to him. This requires the carer to be flexible in her approach, and to expect variations in patient dependency. In this sense, nursing care involves dealing with unexpected demands from the patient. The use of problem-solving skills means that carers need to be well educated in the dynamics of human interaction, especially in communication and counselling skills.

Peplau's model of nursing gives us the opportunity to use an important interpersonal tool. It has been a model for our consideration for some time now, and it still has the flexibility to be used in today's world of nursing. It can realistically be used in a variety of disciplines in nursing; as with some other nursing models, its value is seen in continual use and repeated assessment of how it can help in providing proficient nursing care.

In striving for excellence, Peplau's model needs to be tested in different settings: it has the potential to reveal to us how we can move forward and grow as a profession.

Aggleton, P. and Chalmers, H. 1990. Nursing models – Peplau's development model. In *Nursing Times*, Vol. 86, No. 2 (January 1990), 38–40.

Altschul, A. T. 1972. *Patient Interaction: a study of interaction patterns in acute psychiatric wards*. Edinburgh: Churchill Livingstone.

Anderson, E. R. 1973. *The Role of the Nurse*. London: Royal College of Nursing.

Benoliel, J. Q. 1977. The interaction between theory and research. In *Nursing Outlook*, Vol. 25, 108–13.

Breakwell, G. M. 1987. Mapping counselling in the non-primary sector of the NHS. In *Report for the British Association for Counselling*.

Chin, R. 1980. The utility of systems models and developmental models for practitioners. In Riehl, J. P. and Roy, C. eds. *Conceptual Models for Nursing Practice*. New York: Appleton-Century-Crofts.

Deane, D. and Campbell, J. 1985. *Developing Professional Effectiveness in Nursing*. Reston, Virginia: Prentice-Hall.

Devito, J. 1989. *The Interpersonal Communication Book*, 5th edn. New York: Harper and Row.

Duck, S. 1986. *Human Relationships – an introduction to social psychology*. London: Sage Publications.

Faulkner, A. 1979. Monitoring nurse–patient conversation in a ward. In *Nursing Times* 75 (Suppl.), 95–6.

Fawcett, J. 1989. *Analysis and Evaluation of Conceptual Models of Nursing*, 2nd edn. Philadelphia: F. A. Davis.

Friedman, H. S. and Dimatteo, M. R. 1982. *Interpersonal Issues in Health Care*. New York: Academic Press.

Hase, S. and Douglas, A. 1986. *Human Dynamics and Nursing*. Edinburgh: Churchill Livingstone.

Heiss, J. 1976. *Family Roles and Interaction*. Chicago: Rand-McNally.

Heiss, J. 1981. *The Social Psychology of Interaction*. Englewood Cliffs, New Jersey: Prentice-Hall.

Jarvinnaan, K. A. J. 1955. Can ward rounds be a danger to patients with myocardial infarction? In *British Medical Journal* (1), 318–20.

Johnston, M. 1976. Communication of patients' feelings in hospitals. In Bennett, A. E. ed. *Communication between Doctors and Patients*. Oxford: Nuffield Provincial Hospitals Trust/Oxford University Press.

Kagan, C. 1985. *Interpersonal Skills in Nursing – research and applications*. Croom Helm.

Knowles, M. S. 1973. *The Modern Practice of Adult Education*. New York: New York University Press.

Malan, D. H. 1979. *Individual Psychotherapy and the Science of Psychodynamics*. London: Butterworth.

Meleis, A. 1985. *Theoretical Nursing: development and progress*. Philadelphia: Lippincott.

Moult, A., Melia, K. and Pembury, S. A. M. 1978. *Patterns of Ward Organisation*. Edinburgh: Nursing Research Unit (unpublished report).

O'Toole, A. W. and Welt, S. R. 1989. *Interpersonal Theory in Nursing Practice: selected works of Hildegard E. Peplau*. New York: Springer.

Peplau, H. E. 1952. *Interpersonal Relations in Nursing*. New York: G. P. Putnam.

Peplau, H. E. 1960, Talking with patients. In *American Journal of Nursing* Vol. 60, No. 7 (July 1960), 964–6.

Peplau, H. E. 1962. Interpersonal techniques: the crux of psychiatric nursing. In *American Journal of Nursing*, Vol. 62, No. 6 (June 1962), 50–4.

Peplau, H. E. 1965. The heart of nursing: interpersonal relations. In *The Canadian Nurse*, Vol. 61, No. 4 (April 1965), 273–5.

Peplau, H. E. 1969. Professional closeness. In *Nursing Forum*, Vol. 8, No. 4, 343–59.

Peplau, H. E. 1971. Process and concept of learning. In Burd, S. F. and Marshall, M. A. eds. *Some Clinical Approaches to Psychiatric Nursing*. London: Macmillan.

Peplau, H. E. 1978. Psychiatric nursing: role of nurses and psychiatric nurses. In *International Nursing Review*, Vol. 25 (2), 41–7.

Peplau, H. E. 1988. *Interpersonal Relations in Nursing*, 2nd edn. Basingstoke: Macmillan.

Stockwell, F. 1972. *The Unpopular Patient*. London: Royal College of Nursing.

Wang, A. M. and Blumberg, P. 1983. A study of interaction techniques of nursing faculty in the clinical area. In *Journal of Nursing Education*, 22, 144–51.

of patient 2
developmental model 93–4
dimensions of maturation 13–14
documentation of nursing
        practice 100–1, 102

elderly patient, care study 52–60
emergency admission, care
        study 61–74
emotional support 36
equilibrium 4
esteem support 36
evaluation of care 101–4
    see also care studies
expert–compliant alliance 38
exploitation phase 12–13
extending questions 16

Faulkner, A. 19
fear, of professionals 39
feelings, and care 33–4, 104
flexibility of approach 32, 104
framework, model as 32–3, 97–8

'growth cues' 12

health 3–4
hearing, *vs.* listening 14
Heiss, J. 94
home, nursing at 36–7
hospital, *vs.* community,
        nursing 36–7
humanistic model, use of 98
hypothetical questions 16

identification phase 11–12
'ill-health hypothesis' 34, 35
illness 3–4
    as learning experience 22
individual, patient as 21, 31, 33,
        37, 94
information:
    from the patient 31
    provision of 23
institutionalisation 38
interaction 93
    see also nurse–patient
    relationship

Jarvinnaan, K. A. J. 39

Johnston, M. 19

Knowles, M. S. 13–14

language skills 15
leader, nurse as 25–6
learning experience:
    illness as 22
    nursing as 20–1
linking/clarifying questions 16
listening skills 14–15

man, nature of 4–5
management styles, health
        care 25
Melia, K. 19
mental health, care studies 75–83,
        83–90
models 1, 93
    functions of 98
Moult, A. 19

needs 5
nurse:
    attitudes, beliefs and values 31
    development of 2
    flexibility 32, 104
    roles of 6–8, 19–28, 94
    self-awareness 2, 32, 104
    support for 100
nurse–patient relationship 1
    development of 7, 10–14
    influences on 9
    phases (*q.v.*) of interaction
        1–2, 94–5
nursing:
    alliance 34–9
    definition of 6
    democratic 25–6
    documentation of practice
        100–1, 102
    as helping patient towards
        health 3
    influences on 9
    as learning experience 20–1, 31
    as nurturing process 4–5
    plan of care 3
    process 22
    roles (*q.v.*) 6–8, 19–28, 94
    social context of 5, 94